Warning and Disclaimer:

Every effort has been made to make this book as complete and as accurate as possible, but no warranty of fitness is implied. The author and the publisher shall have neither liability nor responsibility to any person or entity with respect to any loss or damages arising from the information contained in this book.

Go Pass - MRCPCH CLINICAL
Authored by Dr Ehab Hanafy
ISBN-13: 9781515246602
ISBN-10: 1515246604

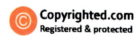

© 2015 Ehab Hanafy All Rights Reserved

No part of this book shall be reproduced, stored in a retrieval system, or transmitted by any means – electronic, mechanical, photocopying, recording, or otherwise – without written permission from the publisher.

to my girls;

Selma, Selene & Rania

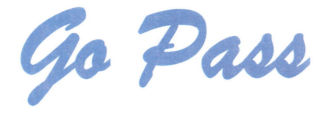

First Edition 2015

MRCPCH

DCH

Pediatric Clinical Examinations

By: Dr. Ehab Hanafy

PREFACE

Go Pass is a quick revision notes and is not considered by any means to be a textbook or a reference book for studying Pediatrics. The optimal benefit from this book will be achieved after a thorough reading in the Pediatric field, training and practicing clinical examination in the real life.

Moreover *Go pass* is recommended to save effort and to have all topics reviewed in short time just before setting your exam.

Once I studied from this note when it looked like this…

So I have done every effort and it took me a long time to achieve it like how it looks like now in order to be at the candidate's convenience and satisfaction.

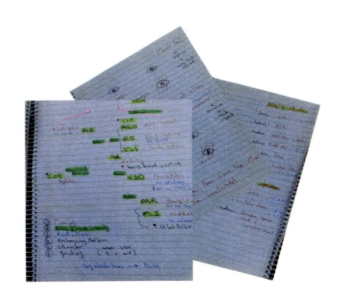

This book is designed as study note which covers all the aspects of the MRCPCH clinical examination and other Pediatric clinical exams. It is also useful for medical students, general practitioners and young pediatricians who are planning to set any pediatric clinical examination.

Go Pass is arranged in 6 main parts

- ✓ Clinical short cases
- ✓ Development assessment
- ✓ Communication skills
- ✓ History taking
- ✓ Review notes
- ✓ ECG notes

Ehab Hanafy

بِسْمِ اللهِ الرَّحْمٰنِ الرَّحِيمِ

وَقُلْ رَبِّ أَدْخِلْنِي مُدْخَلَ صِدْقٍ وَأَخْرِجْنِي مُخْرَجَ صِدْقٍ وَاجْعَلْ لِي مِنْ لَدُنْكَ سُلْطَانًا نَصِيرًا
(سورة الاسراء اية:80)

And say, "My Lord, cause me to enter a sound entrance and to exit a sound exit and grant me from Yourself a supporting authority."

GET STARTED RIGHT AWAY

- Wash your hands
- Roll up long sleeved shirt

LOOK GREAT EVERY TIME

- Introduction, patient identification and consent
- Establish rapport with the child and parents
- Ensure privacy, undress the child
- Positioning

Confidence — Trust — Examine

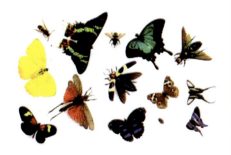

GIVE IT THAT FINISHING TOUCH

HOW TO APPROACH

1. *Again and again, first step is to introduce yourself to the parent and child, and establish a rapport.*
2. *Take a consent from the parent to conduct your clinical examination.*
3. *Ensure that you wash your hands between cases and show the examiner that you are keen to do so.*
4. *During examination always ask for the child's permission before attempting any action and always ask the child if he or she has any pain.*
5. *In 9 out of 10 stations you will be given an instruction which you have to fully concentrate because it may simply carry the key to your success.*
6. *You may be asked to do a running commentary or to perform your examination then to comment at the end.*
7. *Make sure that you finish as early as you can, time management may be the reason of failure, so don't only master the technique but master the timing and target it to 6 minutes maximum.*
8. *Try to pick the findings as much as you can then interpret them in your mind while examining.*
9. *At the end, suggest to conduct further examination to other related systems if applicable.*
10. *Suggest a provisional diagnosis, and probably you will be asked about differentials, finally, Suggest a management plan.*

Contents

Clinical short cases — 4

- Cardiovascular Examination — 5
- Abdominal Examination — 8
- Nutritional Assessment — 11
- Respiratory Examination — 12
- Neurology Examination
  - Cranial Nerve Examination — 15
  - Eye Examination — 16
  - CNS Examination — 17
- Musculoskeletal Examination — 24
  - PGALS — 25
  - Specific Joint Examination — 27
  - Hand and Wrist Examination — 29
- Approach to Short Stature — 30
- Approach to Tall Stature — 33
- Thyroid Examination — 34

Development Assessment — 38

Communication Skills — 45

History Taking — 52

Reviews — 59

ECG — 224

Clinical Short Cases

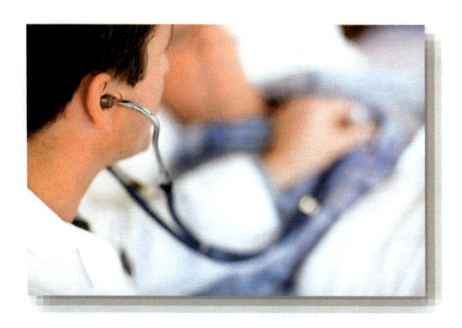

Cardiovascular Examination

General:

1. Wellbeing
2. Alertness and Consciousness
3. Plotting weight and height on the growth charts
4. Dysmorphic features if any
5. Color
6. Surrounding environment; monitors, O2 supply, Work of breathing

Hands and Arms:

1. Warm or Cold hands
2. Clubbing or not
3. Stigmata of endocarditis; Osler's nodules, Janeway lesions, Splinter hemorrhage
4. Peripheral Cyanosis
5. Pulse; Rate, Rhythm, Volume, Character, Symmetry, Femoral Pulse (normal or week), Radio-femoral delay
6. Blood Pressure

Head and Neck:

1. Conjunctival Pallor
2. Conjunctival Jaundice
3. Central Cyanosis
4. Dental Hygiene
5. Jugular venous pressure
6. Carotid Pulsations

Finger clubbing

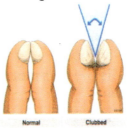

Normal values

PULSE/min	AGE (y)	BP (S)
110-150	1	70-90
80-120	2	80-100
70-110	5	90-110
60-100	8	100-120

Cyanosis

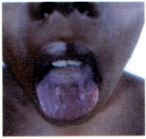

Osler's nodules

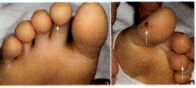

Splinter hemorrhage

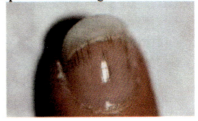

Chest:

Inspection:
1. Shape
2. Symmetry
3. Scars
4. Scoliosis
5. Visible Pulsations

Palpation:
- Apex; site, character, right ventricular heave
- Thrills; carotid, suprasternal, upper left and right sternal edge

Auscultation: (heart sounds, murmurs, additional sounds)
- Pulmonary area
- Aortic area
- Tricuspid area
- Along sternal edge
- Mitral area
- Back side
- Lung bases

Abdomen:

1. Hepatomegaly
2. Splenomegaly
3. Ascites
4. Situs inversus
5. Scars

Groin:

1. Scars; catheterization, central lines
2. Femoral Pulse

At the end I would like to check the:
- ✓ Growth charts
- ✓ Blood pressure
- ✓ JVP
- ✓ Peripheral and sacral edema
- ✓ Fundoscopy and urine dipstick

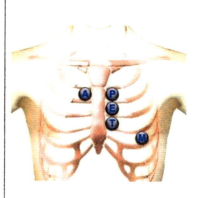

S1 loud: fever, anemia, excitation
S2 loud: Pulmonary Hypertension

S2:
Widely split: ASD, PS
Fixed Split: ASD
Single S2: Pulmonary Hypertension, Severe PS, AS, Pulmonary Atresia
Reverse split: Severe AS

Aortic click over LLSE
Pulmonary Click over ULSE

MURMURS; comment on:
1. Timing
2. Site of maximum intensity
3. Radiation
4. Enhancing position
5. Grading (with thrill (3), no thrill (4-5)

Murmurs

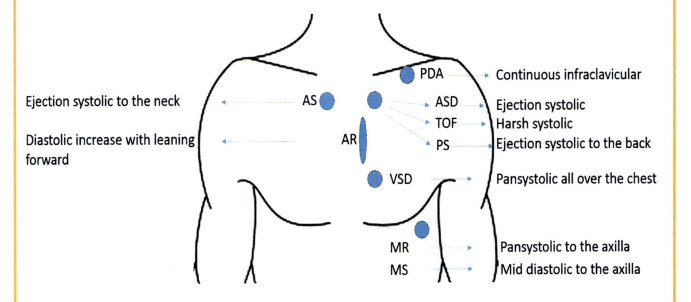

Scenarios

PINK	PINK with Operation
VSD ASD PDA AS PS AR MR INNOCENT murmur	Lateral thoracotomy + absent Radial pulse: COA Lateral thoracotomy: PDA Median sternotomy: anything as pink Median and Lateral thoracotomy: TOF Median and Lateral + absent radial pulse: complex CHD
CYANOSED	**CYANOSED with Operation**
TOF Eisenmenger: older ages, Down syndrome, Loud P2, Clubbing, Murmur	Lateral: TOF with its murmur Lateral: Pulmonary atresia with single S2, absent Radial Median: complex Cyanotic CHD

Abdominal Examination

General:

1. Wellbeing
2. Alertness and Consciousness
3. Plotting weight and height on the growth charts
4. Dysmorphic features if any
5. Color
6. Surrounding environment; monitors, NGT, Cannulas

Hands and Arms:

1. Warm or Cold hands
2. Clubbing or not
3. Koilonychias
4. Palmar erythema
5. Pulse
6. Blood Pressure

Head and Neck:

1. Conjunctival Pallor
2. Conjunctival Jaundice
3. Blue Sclera
4. Dental Hygiene
5. Mouth pigmentation
6. Mouth ulceration
7. Stomatitis, large tongue
8. Jugular venous pressure

Koilonychias

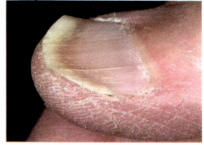

Palmer Erythema

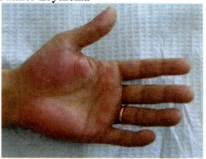

Peutz-Jeghers syndrome

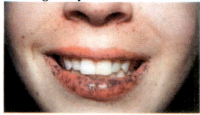

Blue Sclera

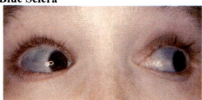

Macroglossia

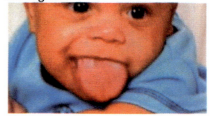

Chest:
1. Shape
2. Symmetry
3. Scars
4. Scoliosis
5. Spider Navei
6. Gynecomastia

Abdomen:
Inspection:
1. Shape; distended, flat, scaphoid
2. Symmetry
3. Scars
4. Abnormal vessels; caput medusa
5. Umbilicus
6. Hernias
7. Genitalia
8. Injection sites

Palpation:
- Superficial, deep, bimanual
- Liver, spleen, kidney, any mass
- Edge, surface, consistency, tenderness

Percussion:
1. Upper edge of the liver
2. Mild splenomegaly
3. Ascites

Auscultation:
1. Bowel sounds
2. Venous hum, right upper quadrant, anastomosis of portal hypertension

Back of Abdomen:
Inspection:
Scoliosis and Gluteal muscle bulk
Palpation:
Tenderness over renal angle and spine
Percussion:
Direct over spinous processes (Spinous process)
Auscultation:
Renal angle bruits

Lower limb edema

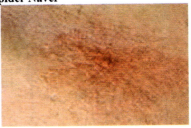
Spider Navei

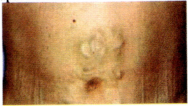
Caput Medusa

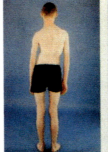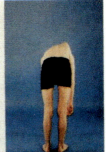
Scoliosis

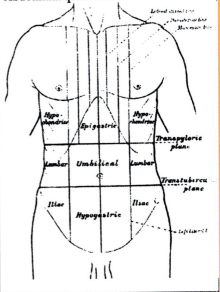
Abdominal quadrants

Abdominal scars

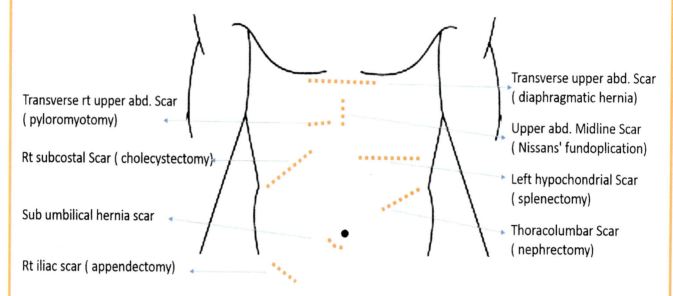

Causes of pelvic masses

- Renal transplant
- Constipation
- Full bladder
- Tumors
- Inflammatory mass (Crohn's disease, appendicitis)

Common Scenarios

Huge Hepatomegaly· **Glycogen Storage Disease**

Hepatomegaly + splenectomy + jaundice: **Chronic Hemolytic Anemia**

Splenomegaly· **full differential diagnosis**

Portal Hypertension (splenomegaly, Ascites, Caput Medusa): **Portal Vein Obstruction**

Portal Hypertension + hepatomegaly· **Congenital Hepatic Fibrosis**

Portal Hypertension + hepatomegaly + liver disease: **Biliary Atresia**

Nutritional Assessment

General:

- Wellbeing
- Alertness and Consciousness
- Dysmorphic features if any
- Color
- Environment; NGT, Gastrostomy

- Plotting weight and height on growth charts

- If there is loss of subcutaneous fat:
  Check the subscapular and triceps skin fold thickness

- If there is loss in muscle bulk:
  Check the mid upper arm circumference

- Examine the mouth
- Examine the nails
- Examine the hair

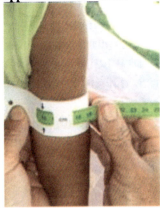

Mid upper arm circumference

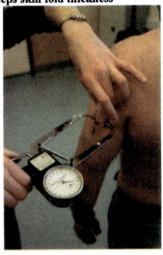

Triceps skin fold thickness

Causes of growth failure

- **Increased loss:** malabsorption
- **Decreased intake:** anorexia, nausea, psychogenic
- **Increased demands:** chronic diseases, Cystic fibrosis, Cerebral Palsy, BDP, CHD, IBD

Recommendations:

- Increase caloric intake
- Administration of food via NGT, Gastrostomy, TPN
- Pancreatic enzymes & Vitamin supplementation

Respiratory Examination

General:

1. Wellbeing
2. Alertness and Consciousness
3. Plotting weight and height on the growth charts
4. Dysmorphic features if any
5. Color
6. Surrounding environment; inhalers, nebulizers, sputum cup, peak flow meter

Hands and Arms:

1. Warm or Cold hands
2. Clubbing or not
3. Peripheral cyanosis
4. Pulse
5. Blood Pressure

Head and Neck:

1. Conjunctival Pallor
2. Central Cyanosis
3. Dental Hygiene
4. Nasal polyps, deviated nasal septum
5. Tonsils, pharynx
6. Jugular Venous Pressure

Nasal polyps

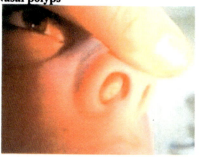

Deviated nasal septum

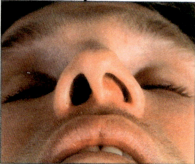

Peripheral cyanosis

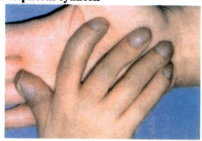

Peak flow meters

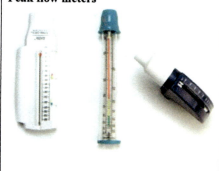

Chest:
Inspection:

1. **S**hape; carinatum, excavatum, Harrison Sulcus
2. **S**ymmetry
3. **S**cars
4. **S**coliosis
5. **S**putum, amount, color, consistency
6. Work of breathing & respiratory distress
   a. Nasal flaring
   b. Sternal recession
   c. Subcostal, intercostal recession
   d. Tracheal tug
   e. Grunting

Palpation:

- Mediastinal position
  - ✓ Apex
  - ✓ Trachea
- Chest expansion; anterior and posterior
- Vocal fremitus
  - ✓ By ulnar border of the hand
  - ✓ Ask to say ninety nine
  - ✓ Increase with consolidation
  - ✓ Decrease with effusion and pneumothorax

Percussion:

1. Anterior
   - ✓ Supra-clavicular
   - ✓ Clavicular
   - ✓ Mammary
   - ✓ Infra-mammary
2. Posterior
   - ✓ Supra-scapular
   - ✓ Inter-scapular
   - ✓ Infra-scapular

- Increased resonance: pneumothorax
- Impaired note: collapse, consolidation
- Stony dullness: pleural effusion

Pectus carinatum

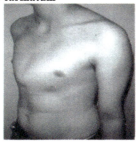

Pectus excavatum

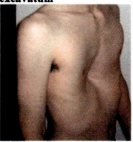

Harrison's Sulcus

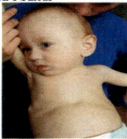

Anterior chest expansion

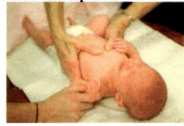

Posterior chest expansion

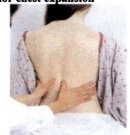

Auscultation:

1. Vesicular or bronchial breathing
2. Air entry & expiratory phase
3. Wheezes, inspiratory or expiratory
4. Crepitation; fine or coarse
5. Vocal resonance
   - ✓ Ask to say ninety nine
   - ✓ Muffled. normal
   - ✓ Clearly heard. consolidation
   - ✓ Markedly reduced. effusion

Others:

1. Palpate for hepatomegaly
2. Check lower limb edema
3. Rule out right side heart failure
4. Growth charts
5. Peak flow meter

Don't forget back auscultation!
Liver palpation
Lower limb edema

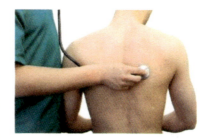

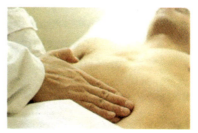

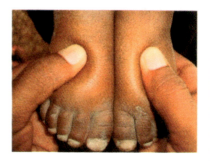

Scenarios

Hyper-expanded chest + clubbing: Cystic fibrosis, Bronchiectasis

Other DD.. empyema, suppurative lung disease, fibrosing alveolitis, TB, primary ciliary dyskinesia

Hyper-expanded chest + No clubbing: Asthma, chronic lung disease

Acute conditions: Pneumonia, effusion

Cranial Nerve Examination

General:
1. Wellbeing
2. Alertness and Consciousness
3. Plotting weight and height on the growth charts
4. Dysmorphic features if any

1 Olfactory nerve:
Do you have any problem with smelling?

2 Optic nerve:
- Visual acuity; ask the child to read in any book
- Visual fields
- Pupillary reflex

3,4,6 Oculomotor, Trochlear, Abducent:
- Eye movement; 8 directions
- Nystagmus
- Ptosis
- Squint

5 Trigeminal:
- Sensation over ophthalmic, maxillary and mandibular spaces
- Motor; palpate temporalis and masseters muscles

7 Facial:
Close eye, raise brows, smile, show teeth, puff cheek

8 Auricular:
Whisper behind the child's ears

9,10 Glossopharyngeal, Vagus:
Do you have any difficulty in swallowing, drooling of saliva, or nasal tone of voice?!

11 Accessory:
- Move face from side to side against resistance
- Move shoulder up against resistance
- Check for sternomastoid and trapezius muscle wasting

12 Hypoglossal:
- Inspect tongue for wasting, fasciculation, deviation
- Move tongue side to side

Visual field
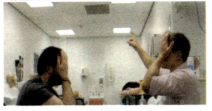

3rd CN palsy
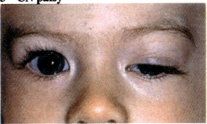

4th CN palsy
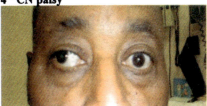

Causes of CN palsies in general:
- Increases ICP
- Trauma
- Infections
- Tumors

Eye Examination

General:

1. Wellbeing
2. Alertness and Consciousness
3. Plotting weight and height on the growth charts
4. Dysmorphic features if any
5. Glasses or not
6. Notice if any·
   - Coloboma
   - Clouding
   - Cataract

Do you have blurred or double vision?

Cranial nerves:

2 Optic nerve:
- Visual acuity; let him read in any book
- Visual fields
- Pupillary reflex

3,4,6 Oculomotor, Trochlear, Abducent:
- Eye movement; 8 directions
- Nystagmus
- Ptosis
- Squint

Others:

- Corneal reflection
- Cover and uncover test
- Fundoscopy

Cataract

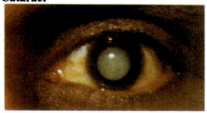

Corneal clouding

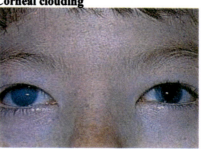

Coloboma

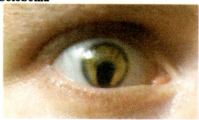

Ptosis

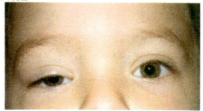

6th CN palsy

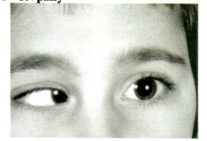

CNS Examination

General:

1. Wellbeing
2. Alertness and Consciousness
3. Plotting weight and height on the growth charts
4. Dysmorphic features if any
5. Environment:
   - Wheel chair
   - Orthosis
   - Braces
   - Catheters
   - Nappies
   - NGT
   - Helmets

Hands and arms:
- Shake hands
- Right or left handed

Head and neck:
1. Size
2. Shape
3. Sutures
4. Shunts
5. Symmetry

CNS:
- Motor
- Sensory
- Cerebellar
- Gait
- Back

Orthosis

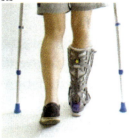

Chest braces

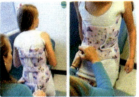

VP shunt

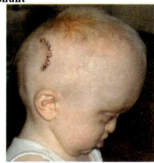

Abnormal head shape

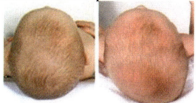

Normal   Plagiocephaly

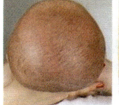 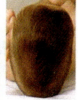

Brachycephaly   Dolichocephaly

Motor examination

Inspection:
1. Posture
2. Muscle bulk; wasted or hypertrophied
3. Involuntary movements:
   - Fasciculation
   - Tremors
   - Chorea
   - Athetosis
   - Tics
4. Scars
5. Contractures or deformities
6. Rashes
7. Swelling

Ask if any pain when you proceed

Tone:
- UL, wrist, elbow, shoulder
- LL; ankle, knee, hip

Clonus:
- Knee, ankle

Reflexes:

1. UL
   - Biceps   C5,C6
   - Supinator   C5,C6
   - Triceps   C6,C7
2. LL
   - Knee   L3,L4
   - Ankle   S1
3. Superficial
   - Abdominal   T7-T12
4. Babinski   S1

Clonus

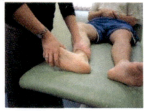

Triceps reflex

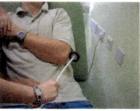

Biceps reflex

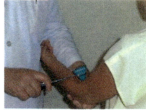

Knee reflex

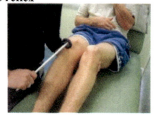

Ankle reflex

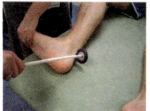

DD of chorea
- CP, Sydenham's chorea
- Huntington's chorea
- Wilson's disease
- Anti-convulsunts side effects

Power:
Upper limb
- Shoulder
  - ✓ Abduction C5,C6
  - ✓ Adduction
  - ✓ Flexion
  - ✓ Extension
- Elbow
  - ✓ Flexion   C5,C6
  - ✓ Extension   C7,C8
- Wrist
  - ✓ Flexion
  - ✓ Extension
- Finger
  - ✓ Flexion   C8
  - ✓ Extension
  - ✓ Abduction   C8,T1
  - ✓ Adduction
- Thumb
  - ✓ Flexion
  - ✓ Extension
  - ✓ Opposition

Lo
- Hip
  - ✓ Flexion   L1
  - ✓ Extension   S3
  - ✓ Abduction
  - ✓ Adduction   L2
- Knee
  - ✓ Flexion   S2
  - ✓ Extension   L4
- Ankle
  - ✓ Planter flexion   S1
  - ✓ Dorsiflexion   L4
- Great toe
  - ✓ Planter flexion
  - ✓ Dorsiflexion

Shoulder abduction and adduction

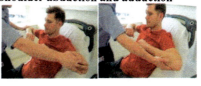

Elbow flexion and extension

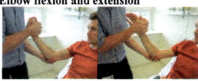

Wrist flexion and extension

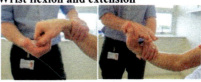

Finger flexion and extension

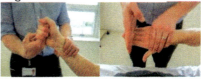

Hip extension and flexion

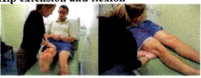

Knee flexion and extension

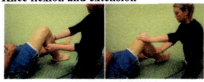

Ankle dorsiflexion and planter flexion

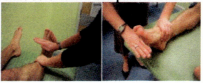

0 No power
1 Traces of contractions
2 Active with gravity eliminated
3 Active against gravity
4 Active against resistance
5 Normal power

Sensory examination

Superficial:

- **Pain** with a pin
- **Light touch** with a cotton
- **Temperature** with a cold tuning fork

From proximal to distal

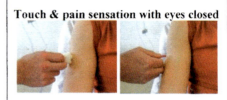
Touch & pain sensation with eyes closed

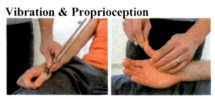
Vibration & Proprioception

Deep:

- **Vibration** with tuning fork
    - ✓ Big toe
    - ✓ Medial malleolus
    - ✓ Knee
    - ✓ Anterior superior iliac spine
    - ✓ Styloid process of radius
    - ✓ Elbow
    - ✓ Shoulder

Distal to proximal
Demonstrate on sternum first

- **Proprioception**
  Hold thumb, big toe, finger up and down

Demonstrate first

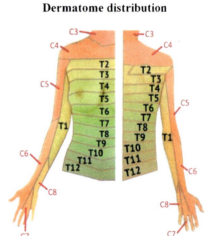
Dermatome distribution

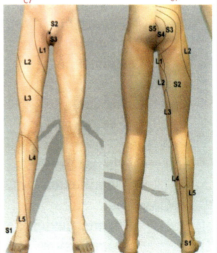

Cortical sensations

Cerebellar system

Head:

- Dysarthria when speaking with him
- Check for nystagmus

Upper limb:

- **Tremors**: stretch your hand
- **Tone**
- **Dysmetria**
  Index to nose, index to my index
- **Dysrhythmia**
  Thumb to all finger tips
- **Dysdiadokokinesia**
  Clap hand back and fro
- **Rebound phenomenon**
  Stretch hands, palm up and pull down while closing child's eye

Lower limb:

- **Tone**
- **Gait**
- **Romberg's test**
- **Heal to heal**

Tremors

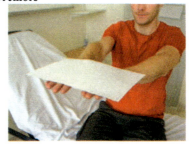

Dysdiadokokinesia

 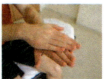

Dysmetria

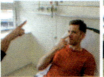 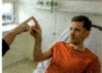

Heal to heal

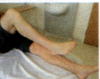 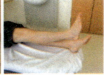

Romberg's test

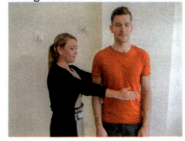

Gait examination

While standing:

- Check for shortened limb
- Position of foot and knee

Ask to:

- Walk forward then come back
- Walk on tiptoe
- Walk on heal
- Walk heal to toe
- Run

Then do:

- Romberg's test
- Gower sign
- Trendelenburg test

Types of gait

- **Hemiplegic**
- **Diplegic**
- **Ataxic**; broad based, staggering, tendency to fall
- **Waddling**; myopathy
- **Steppage**; neuropathy, foot drop
- **Shuffling**; parkinsonism

- **Trendelenburg**;
  Non painful limb
  Congenital hip dysplasia
  Muscle dystrophy
- **Antalgic**
  Painful limb
  Infection
  Trauma
  Perthes disease

Gower sign

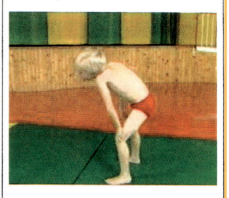

Trendelenburg test

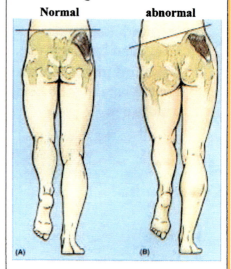

Common scenarios:

Cerebral Palsy
Neuromuscular diseases
Ataxia
- Ataxia telangiectasia
- Friedreich's ataxia
- Ataxic CP

Neurocutaneous syndromes
- Neurofibromatosis
- Tuber sclerosis
- Sturge Weber
- Incontinenta Pigmenti

Neuromuscular disease

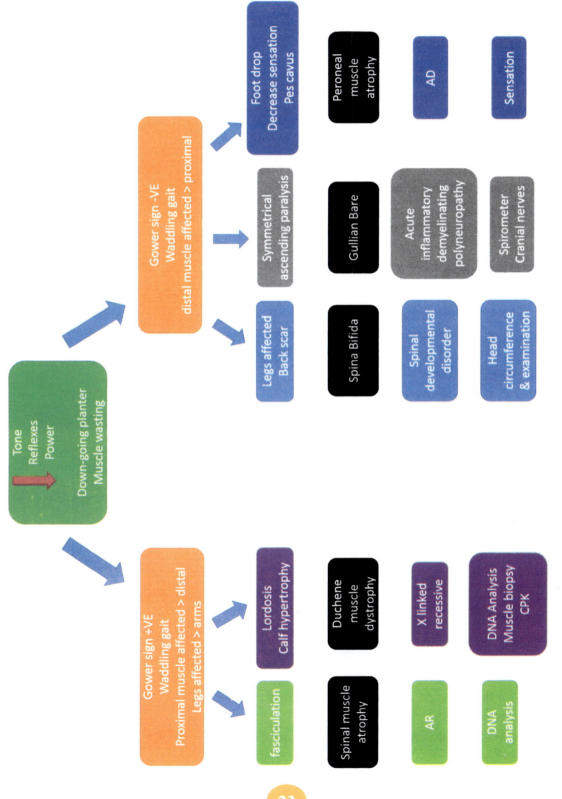

Musculoskeletal Examination

While you are examining a single joint or the whole skeletal system or even PGALS examination there should be an initial **common pathway** to start with.

Overview

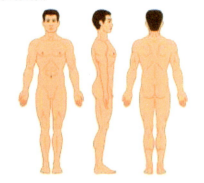

1- General:
1. Wellbeing
2. Alertness and Consciousness
3. Plotting weight and height on the growth charts
4. Dysmorphic features if any
5. Environment:
   - Wheel chair, Orthosis, Braces, splints

2- Body Overview:
- **Front**
  - ✓ Elbow extension
  - ✓ Quadriceps bulk and symmetry
  - ✓ Forefoot abnormalities
- **Back**
  - ✓ Shoulder bulk and symmetry
  - ✓ Spine alignment
  - ✓ Gluteal bulk and symmetry
  - ✓ Popliteal swellings
  - ✓ Calf muscle bulk and symmetry
  - ✓ Hind foot abnormalities
- **Sides**
  - ✓ Cervical lordosis
  - ✓ Thoracic kyphosis
  - ✓ Lumbar lordosis
  - ✓ Knee flexion/hyperextension

Kyphosis / lordosis

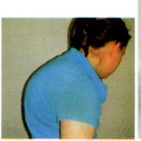
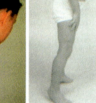

Genu varum   Genu valgum

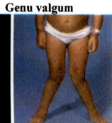

3- Screening questions:
1. Do you have any pain or difficulty in moving your arms, legs, neck or back?
2. When you get dressed, are you able to do this yourself without any help?
3. Can you walk up and down the stairs without any problems?

Intoeing

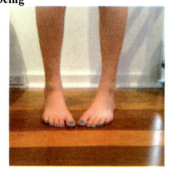

PGALS examination - common pathway +

Gait:

1. Observe the patient walking.
2. *Walk on your heels.*
3. *Walk on your tip-toes.*

Arms:

1. *Put your hands out in front of you.*
2. *Turn your hand over and make a fist.*
3. *Pinch your thumb and index together*
4. *Touch the tips of your fingers.*
5. Squeeze MCPJs.
6. *Put your hands and wrists together*
7. *Put your hands back to back.*
8. *Reach up as far as you can.*
9. *Look at the ceiling.*
10. *Put your hands behind your neck.*
11. *Place your ear on your shoulder*
12. *Open your mouth wide and place 3 fingers inside.*

Legs:

1. Feel for effusion at the knee.
2. *Bring your ankle up to your bottom.*
3. Passive movement of hip and knee including rotation of hip.

Spine:

1. Observe curvature of spine from the sides and behind.
2. *Bend forwards.*

Indications of PGALS:

1. General instruction: examine MSK system
2. History of pain or joint stiffness
3. Suspect systemic condition affecting the joints
4. You find a joint problem

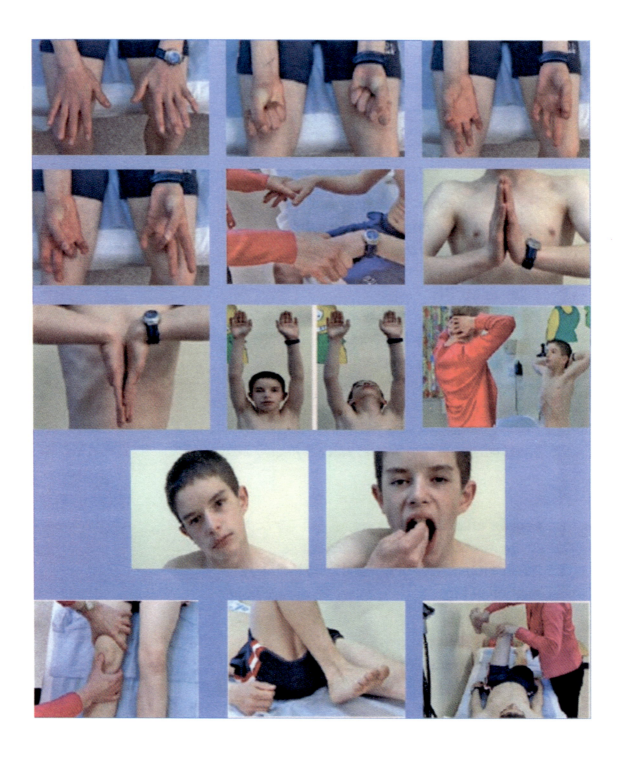

Specific joint examination - common pathway +

Look: **front, back & sides**
1. Posture
2. Symmetry
3. Swelling
4. Scars
5. Rashes
6. Muscle bulk
7. Deformities

Feel:
1. **Temperature**: with back of your fingers then compare
2. **Palpate** the joint space and margins
3. Feel any **tenderness, swellings**
4. On knee examination do:
   - ✓ Bulge test
   - ✓ Patellar tap

Move: *see next page*
1. Assess passive and active movement
2. Ask if there is any pain or stiffness at each point of examination
3. Ask the child to stand when examining the hip, knee and ankle joints

Function:
- **Elbow**: ask the child to touch mouth and nose with hand
- **Shoulder**: ask to put hand behind head and behind back
- **Hip, knee, ankle**: ask the child to walk
- **Spine**: gait, reflexes, lower limb neurologic examination

PGALS: If you want to screen other joints

Relevant systemic examination: Skin, Nails, Eye, CVS, CNS, Abdomen.

Move

Elbow	Shoulder	Head & Neck
Flexion	Flexion	Flexion
Extension	Extension	Extension
Pronation	Abduction	Lateral flexion
Supination	Adduction	Rotation
	External rotation	
	Internal rotation	

Hip	Knee	Ankle & Foot
Flexion	Flexion	Dorsiflexion
Extension	Extension	Plantar flexion
Abduction		Inversion
Adduction		Eversion
• Thomas test	• Anterior, posterior draw test	Toe extension
• Trendelenburg		Toe flexion
• Gower test	• Collateral ligament test	

Spine: Cervical . Thoracic . Lumbosacral

Flexion
Extension
Lateral flexion
Rotation

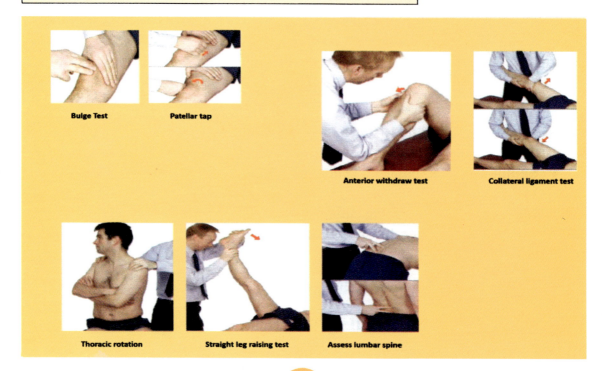

Bulge Test — Patellar tap — Anterior withdraw test — Collateral ligament test

Thoracic rotation — Straight leg raising test — Assess lumbar spine

Hand and Wrist Examination - common pathway +

Look: front, back & sides
1. **Posture**: claw hands, hemiplegia, wrist drop, ulnar deviation
2. **Symmetry**
3. **Swelling**: wrist, PIP, DIP, MPJ
4. **Scars**
5. **Rashes**
6. **Muscle bulk**: thenar, hypothenar muscles
7. **Deformities**. arachynodactyly, syndactyly, polydactyly, clinodactyly, short 4th, 5th metacarpal bones, acromegaly
8. **Nails**: clubbing, koilonychias, pits, onycholysis, white bands
9. **Stigmata of**: endocarditis, liver failure

Feel:
1. Radial pulse
2. Sensation. thenar, hypothenar, web space
3. Temperature
4. **Squeeze**: metacarpal bones
5. **Bimanually examine**: wrist, MPJ
6. **Encircle**: IPJ with index and thumb of both hands

Move:
1. Wrist flexion & extension
2. *Make a fist*
3. *Make a star*
4. *Make a circle with thumb and index*
5. *Touch tips of finger with thumb*

Function:
- Grip strength
- Hold spoon, cup
- Write with pencil

PGALS

Relevant systemic examination

Claw hands
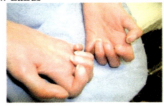

Wrist drop
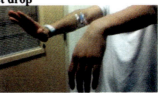

Ulnar deviation
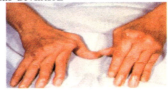

Short 4th, 5th metacarpal bones
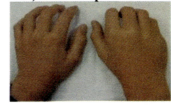

Pitting & onycholysis in psoriasis
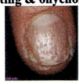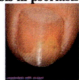

Bimanual examination
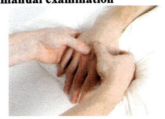

Approach to Short Stature

General:

1. Wellbeing
2. Alertness and Consciousness
3. Plotting weight and height on the growth charts
   + **Measurements**
4. Dysmorphic features if any
5. Environment:
   - Wheel chair, Orthosis, Braces, splints

Hands and arms:

1. Warm or cold
2. Clubbing
3. Nails
4. Joints
5. Pulse
6. Blood pressure
   + **Manoeuvers**

Head and neck:

1. Shape
2. Dysmorphic features
3. Eye; jaundice, corneal clouding, cataract, hypertelorism
4. Nose; nasal septum, nasal bridge
5. Mouth, teeth, palate, angle of mouth
6. Ears; prominent, deformed, auricular tags, glue ear
7. Mandible
8. Neck; deformed, springle deformity, webbed neck

Measurements:

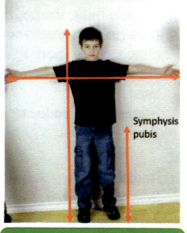

- Height
- Lower segment: From symphysis pubis to floor
- Arm span: Between tips of middle fingers in both sides
- Mid-parental height
  $M = [\text{father height} + (\text{mother} + 12.5)]/2$
  $F = [(\text{father height} - 12.5) + \text{mother}]/2$
- Weight for height
- Head circumference

Manoeuvers

Carrying angle | Deformities

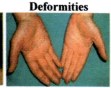

4th, 5th metacarpals | Symmetry

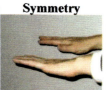

Chest	CVS	Abdomen	Spine	Others
Shape	BP	Obesity	Scoliosis	*Look*
Symmetry		Striae	Lordosis	*next*
Scars		Hernia	Kyphosis	*page*
Nipple		HSM	Deformity	
Axillary hair				

Go Pass – MRCPCH Clinical — Ehab Hanafy

Scenarios

	GH deficiency	Turner	Noonan	Russell Silver
Hands / arms	Small hands and feet	• Natal edema • Hypo plastic nails • Short 4th, 5th MC bones • Wide carrying angle • Pulse	Wide carrying angle	• Hemi hypertrophy • Asymmetry • Clinodactyly • Camptodactyly • Syndactyly
Head/ neck	Crowding of the face	• Low post. Hair line • Webbed neck • High arched palate • Prominent ears • Glue ear	• Antemongloid slant • Hypertelorism • Webbed neck • Low-set ears • Micrognathia	• Small face • Triangular face • High forehead • Blue sclera • Down-turned mouth corner • Springle neck deformity • Late closure of anterior fontanel
Chest		• Shield chest • Spaced nipples • Scars • Axillary hair	• Shield chest • Spaced nipples	
CVS		Full CVS ex. BP	Full CVS ex.	
Abd.	Central obesity			
Spine				
Other		Develop. Ex. Pubertal staging Audiology	Develop. Ex. Pubertal staging Hematology	Develop. Ex. Pubertal staging Renal ex. Bone age X-ray Genetic tests

4th and 5th metal

	Mucopolysaccharidosis	Achondroplasia	Cushing	Hypothyroidism
Hands/arms	Joint stiffness	• Short broad hands • Ligament laxity • Rhizomelic shortening	Proximal myopathy	
Head/neck	• Corneal clouding • Nasal discharge • Upper airway obstruction • Coarse facies • Thick lips • Flat mid-face • Macrocephaly	• Frontal bossing • Flat nasal bridge • Large head • Prognathism	• Moon face • Acne • Hirsutism • Cataract	• Jaundice • Large tongue • Delayed dentition • Wide fontanel
Chest				
CVS	Congestive heart failure	Full CVS ex.		
Abd.	Hernias HSM		• Buffalo hump • Stria • Scars • Masses	• Constipation • Hernias
Spine	• Kyphosis • Scoliosis	• Lordosis • Scoliosis		
Other	Develop. Ex.	Develop. Ex. Audiology	Develop. Ex. Pubertal staging	Develop. Ex. Pubertal staging

Short + underweight + ill = Cystic fibrosis, coeliac, IBD, BPD, DM

Short + well or obese = Cushing, hypothyroidism, GH deficiency

Short + dysmorphic = Syndromic

Approach to Tall Stature

General:
1. Wellbeing
2. Alertness and Consciousness
3. Plotting weight and height on the growth charts
   + **Measurements**
4. Dysmorphic features if any
5. If there is any thyroid sign, then examine **thyroid gland**
6. Environment:
   - Wheel chair, Orthosis, Braces, splints

Hands and Arms:
1. Warm or Cold hands
2. Hyperthyroid features, then examine **thyroid gland**
3. Arachynodactyly
4. **Beighton score**
5. Pulse
6. Blood Pressure

Head and Neck:
1. High arched palate
2. Thyroid eye signs, then examine **thyroid gland**
3. Goiter, then examine **thyroid gland**

Chest:
1. Shape
2. Symmetry
3. Scars
4. Breast development
5. Signs of puberty

CVS:
If Marfan is suspected

Spine:
Kyphosis or scoliosis

Marfan:
- Examine CVS
- Fundoscopy

Homocystinurea:
- Development assessment
- Fundoscopy

Kleinfelter:
- Examine genital organs
- Pubertal staging

Thyroid:
- Examine reflexes
- Pubertal staging

Beighton score

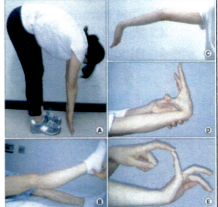

A = 1 point if hand touch floor
B = 1 point for each leg if there is hyperextension at knee
C = 1 point for each arm if wide carrying angle
D = 1 point for each hand
E = 1 point for each hand

A total of 9 points
Hypermobility is suspected for score > 4

Causes of Hemi-Hypertrophy
- Wilm's tumor
- Beckwith Weidman Syndrome
- Russell Silver Syndrome
- Neurofibromatosis (regional overgrowth)
- Lymphangioma (regional overgrowth)
- Hemangioma (regional overgrowth)

Thyroid Examination

General:

1. Wellbeing
2. Alertness and Consciousness
3. Plotting weight and height on the growth charts
4. Dysmorphic features if any

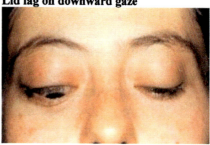
Lid lag on downward gaze

Hands and Arms:

1. Warm or Cold hands
2. Clubbing
3. Fine tremors (extend both hands)
4. Pulse
5. Blood Pressure

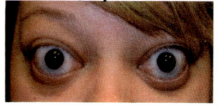
Lid retraction, Proptosis

Head and Neck:

Eye signs

1. Lid edema
2. Lid lag
3. Lid retraction
4. Exophthalmos
5. External ophthalmoplegia

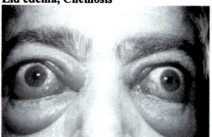
Lid edema, Chemosis

Neck examination: *see next page*

Others:

1. Examine reflexes (slow in hypothyroidism)
2. Proximal myopathy (in hyperthyroidism)
3. Pubertal staging
4. Developmental assessment

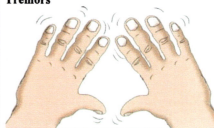
Tremors

Neck examination

Inspection:

1. From front when neck extended
2. Comment on any scars
3. Ask the patient to drink
4. Ask the patient to stick tongue out
5. Examine the tongue for thyroglossal cyst

Palpation:

1. From behind
2. Comment on any swelling; size, shape, surface, consistency
3. Ask the patient to drink
4. Examine the cervical lymph nodes

Percussion:

Percuss the sternum for retrosternal extension

Auscultation:

Any mass for a bruit

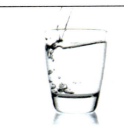

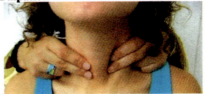

Palpation

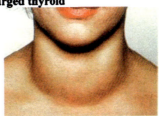

Enlarged thyroid

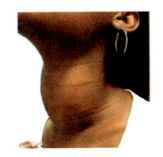

Neck lumps	Goiter		
Thyroglossal cyst Cystic hygroma Branchial cyst Sternomastoid tumors Hemangioma Lymphadenopathy Goiter	Hyperthyroid	Euthyroid	Hypothyroid
	Graves' disease	Autoimmune thyroiditis Iodine deficiency Dyshormonogenesis	
		Colloid goiter	Infiltration Carcinoma

To pass the clinical short cases

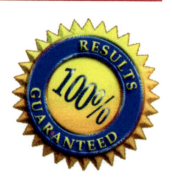

Conduct of examination

- *You have to demonstrate full greeting and introduction to the parents and the child.*
- *Show an appropriate level of confidence.*
- *Be stable and do not rush to the clinical examination.*
- *Put the child at ease.*
- *You should talk and explain examination to child when appropriate.*

Clinical Examination

- *Train and never get bored to get a well-structured and systematic examination.*
- *Master the technique, and do not leave that to the day of the exam.*
- *Correctly identify and interpret clinical signs that you are sure of them.*
- *Displays overall clinical competence.*

Discussion with examiners

- *Suggest a correct differential diagnosis.*
- *Suggests appropriate investigation and management.*
- *Suggest further steps if examination incomplete or inconclusive.*
- *Show understanding to the implications of findings for child and family.*

Common critical errors

- *Poor approach and adherence to infection control.*

- *Approach is not satisfactory in important area or on frequent occasions.*

- *Poor explanation to child and parents.*

- *Poor instructions to child.*

- *Failure of engagement with the child.*

- *Missing several important clinical signs.*

- *Incorrect interpretation of existing clinical signs.*

- *Slow, uncertain unstructured, unsystematic examination.*

- *Poor technique.*

- *Rush through examination.*

- *Describing non-existent findings.*

- *Errors suggesting poor understanding or lack of knowledge with significant clinical implications.*

- *Confident and wrong.*

- *Poor time management.*

- *Leaving no time for discussion.*

- *Too much arguments with the examiners.*

Development Assessment

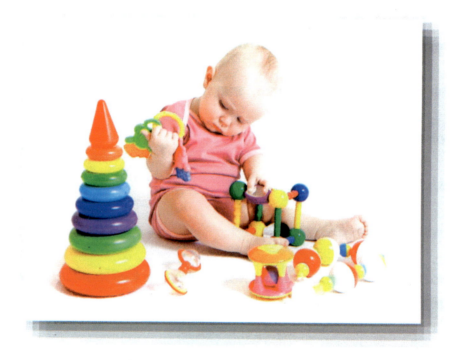

Development Assessment

General:

1. Wellbeing
2. Alertness and Consciousness
3. Plotting weight and height on the growth charts
4. Dysmorphic features if any
5. Environment: (wheel chair, hearing aids, and glasses)

Common phrases:

- *Today the child demonstrates ...., In addition, he could not demonstrate .*
- *When (supine, prone, pull to sit, sits, stands), he/she ... .*
- *For (gross motor, fine & vision, social, speech & hearing) development, this gives him/her developmental age of   .. ..*
- *At the end I would like to formally test for ..   ..*

When:

- Supine
    - Check vision by moving a toy or brick in front of eyes
    - Make a sound at level and below level of both ears
    - Check his head and limb position
    - Give a toy or brick to him/her
    - Give a bead to him/her
    - Wave to him/her
    - Call his/her name
- On side
- Prone
- Ventral
- Pull to sit
- Sitting
- Standing

During this: comment on head position, trunk (ext. or flex), hip (ext. or flex), lower limb and upper limb

Notice startling with noise, Notice social smile, stranger awareness, Listen to his/her own words

Infant Development

Gross Motor

When	Demonstrates	Age
Supine	Head on one side	6 weeks
	Strong kick	3 months
	Elevates head	6 months
Ventral	Head at level of body	6 weeks
	Head above level of body	3 months
	Protective extension	6 months
Prone	Hands off sometimes	6 weeks
	Torso off sometimes	3 months
	Weight bearing on hands	6 months
On side	Rolling	6-7 months
Pull to sit	Head lag	6 weeks
	No head lag	3 months
	Elevates head when about to pull	6 months
Sit	Sits supported	4-6 months
	Straight back/ sits unsupported	6 months
	Sits unsupported (well balanced)	9 months
	Sits from lying	12 months
Stand	Stands supported (LL extended)	6 months
	Stands supported / Crawl	9 months
	Cruise	7-12 months
	Stands alone	12 months
	Walks	12 months

Weight bears on arms 6 months

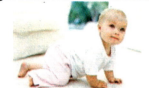

Sits unsupported 6 months

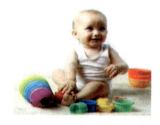

Rolling 7 months

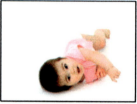

Crawl 9 months

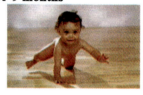

Cruise 10 months

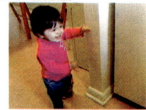

Stand from sitting 12 months

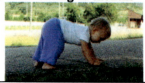

Fine Motor & vision

Demonstrates	Age
Fix and follow 90 degree	6 weeks
Fix and follow 180 degree	3 months
Reaches a brick or toy	3 months
Gets or holds a brick or toy	3-6 months
Mouthing	4 months
Moves a brick or toy from hand to hand	6 months
Points to a bead	6-9 months
Pincer grasp	9-12 months
Points with index	12 months

Social

Demonstrates	Age
Smiles	6 weeks
Stranger awareness	6 months
Peek a poo	9 months
Clap hands or wave	12 months

Hearing & Speech

Demonstrates	Age
Startle at loud voice	6 weeks
Turn to sound	3 months
Bubbling	6 months
Mama / Dada (not specified)	6-9 months
Mama / Dada (specified)	9-12 months
Respond to his name	12 months
1st word (not Mama, Dada)	12-15 months

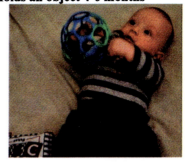

Holds an object 4-6 months

Mouthing 4 months

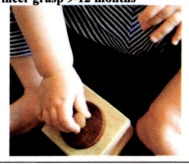

Pincer grasp 9-12 months

Newborn reflexes

MORO	When the baby is startled by a movement, he throws back his head, extends out the arms and legs, cries, then pulls the arms and legs back in
Rooting	The baby will turn his head and open his mouth when the corner of the baby's mouth is stroked
Tonic neck	When a baby's head is turned to one side, the arm on that side stretches out and the opposite arm bends up at the elbow
Stepping	The baby appears to take steps or dance when held upright with his feet touching a solid surface
Grasp	Stroking the palm of a baby's hand causes the baby to close his fingers in a grasp
Suckling	When the roof of the baby's mouth is touched, the baby will begin to suck

Older Child Development

Gross Motor

When	Demonstrates	Age in years
Stands	On tip toe	2
	Squats and stands	2
	On one foot	3
Walk	Carrying toy	1.5
	On tip toe	3
Run	Normal	1.5
	Fast with less control in start and stop	3
	Fast with control in start and stop	4
Climb	Chair	1.5
	Crawls on stairs	1.5
	2 feet/step	2
	1 foot/step	3
	Down 2 feet/step	3
	Up and down	4
Jump	Up	2
	On both feet	3
	Up, down and forward	4
Tricycle		3
Ball	Kicks	2
	Runs to kick	4
	Throws with both hands + body help	2
	Throws with one hand + body rotation	3
	Throws with one hand more mature	4
	Catches with hand & arm (one unit)	2
	Catches with hand & flexed elbow	3
	Catches with hand	4
	Catches and anticipates the ball movement	5

- Demonstrate (stand, walk, run, stand on one foot, tricycle, play with a ball).
- If there is stairs ask to climb, if not ask parent about it.

Crawl on stairs 1.5 years

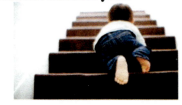

Kick a ball 2 years

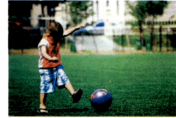

Ride tricycle 3 years

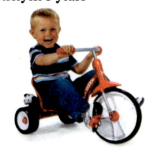

Fast run 3-4 years

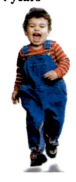

Fine motor & Vision

With	Demonstrates	Age in years
Beads	Pincer grasp	1
	Put in bottle	2
	Thread	3
Book	Browses	1.5
	Show interest in pictures	1.5
	Browses 1 page at a time	2-3
Scissors	Paper cutting	3

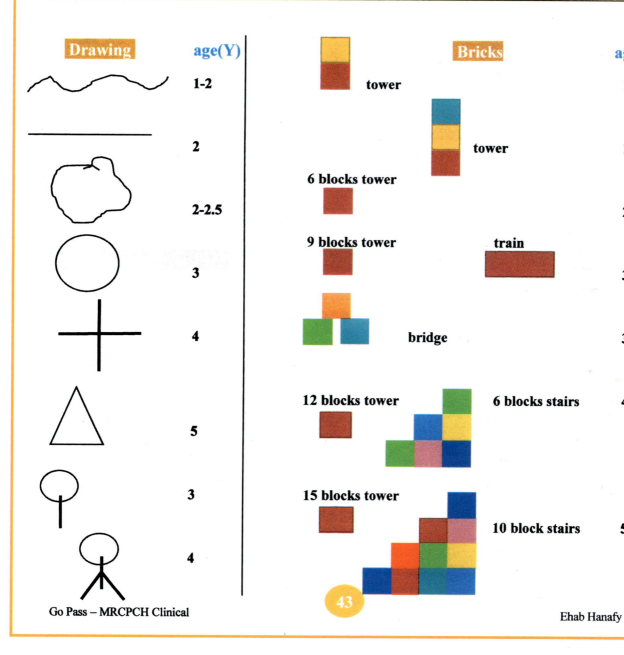

Hearing and speech

When	Demonstrates	Age in years
Name/age/sex	Responds to name	1
	Tells name	2
	Full name	4
	Age	3
	Sex	3
Questions	Where is …….	1.5
	What color is this	3
	What is this .. ..?(shape)	4
Instructions	Show me your (any body part)	1.5
	2 steps instructions	2
	3 steps instructions	3
Words	3	1.5
	20	2
	50	3
	2 words together	2
	4 words together	3
	Counts 1 to 10	4
Conversations	Constant bubbling	1.5
	Can be understood	3
	Grammatical, past & future stories	4
	Fluent	5

Social: mostly history taking

When	Demonstrates	Age in years
Dress	Helps in dressing	12-13 months
	Takes off shoes	15 months
	Dress with little help	2.5-3.5
	Dress alone	3.5-5
Toilet	Toilet need	1.5
	Dry by day	2.5-3
	Alone	3
Eating	Drinks with cup	15 months
	Uses spoon	1.5
	Uses fork & knife	4
Playing	Imitates adults	2
	Plays alone	2.5
	Helps adult	3
	Imaginative play	3
	Shares toys	4
	Chooses friends	5

Communication Skills

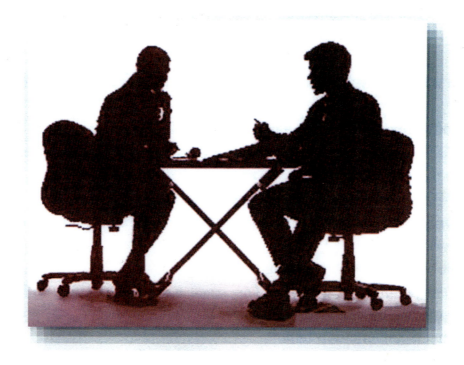

Common scenarios

1. Consent
2. Explaining new treatment
3. Breaking bad news
4. Talking about a medical error
5. Talking to non-compliant adolescent
6. Talking about an ethical issue

Important points to consider:

- Ensure privacy and confidentiality
- Ask open ended questions
- Encourage both parents and child to participate in the conversation
- Include the parents and the child in problem solving
- Boosting parent and child self-esteem
- Be non-judgmental
- Never forget the child's name and age!

The way through any conversation should include 5 main parts:

1- Introduction/clarify roles, agree aims and objectives
- *Good morning Mrs.…. , my name is Dr Ehab and I am the specialist trainee in the team looking after   ., I need to talk to you because   ..*
- *Do you want anyone to be attending with you?*
- *I assure the privacy of this conversation and will do my best so that no one will interrupt us.*

2- Parent or child understanding
- *First of all, can you tell me how much have been already explained to you regarding the current situation*

3- The main conversation bulk

4- Chance for parent or child questions and concerns

5- Summary
- *Mrs. …. I realize that I have given you a lot of information, the main things I want you to remember are*

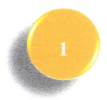

Consent

1- **Introduction/clarify roles, agree aims and objectives**
2- **Parent or child understanding**
3- **The main conversation bulk**
   - Need for the procedure
   - How is it done?
   - Anticipated outcome
   - Any risks and how it will be minimized or dealt with
   - Any other alternatives
4- **Chance for parent or child questions and concerns**
5- **Summary**
   - *Mrs. .. .. I realize that I have given you a lot of information, the main things I want you to remember are.. .. .**can I have your permission on that?!***

NB. Refusal to consent: tell her
If you don't want to go further I think it would be necessary to seek legal advice from authorized facilities and medical protection society.

Explaining new treatment

1- **Introduction/clarify roles, agree aims and objectives**
2- **Parent or child understanding**
3- **The main conversation bulk**
   - What is the new treatment and how it works
   - How is it administered
   - Effectiveness and anticipated outcome
   - Duration and management plan
   - Side effects, how to realize, what to do
4- **Chance for parent or child questions and concerns**
5- **Summary**

Breaking bad news

1. Introduction/clarify roles, agree aims and objectives
2. Parent or child understanding
3. The main conversation bulk

   - Break the new information
   - Implication of this information
   - Give chance to respond, express feelings and ask in mutual conversation
   - Answer honestly
   - Tell what is going to happen next
   - Others

   > ✓ What I am going to do is talk to the team looking after ., and arrange another meeting.
   > ✓ You can write down all your questions and concerns so we can discuss in details.
   > ✓ I will also try to provide you with some patient information and some contact details which perhaps will be useful for you.
   > ✓ I will also arrange a meeting so you can discuss things with our social workers and health educators.

4. Chance for parent or child questions and concerns
5. Summary

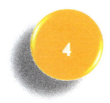

Talking about a medical error

1- **Introduction/clarify roles, agree aims and objectives**
2- **Parent or child understanding**
3- **The main conversation bulk**

- *I need to talk to you to explain about a mistake that was made by ....with regards to.. condition.*
- Tell what happened directly
- Apologize sincerely
- *All the staff in the unit are truly sorry for what has happened*
- Stay calm and show respect
- Explain what are the risks to the child
- What harm has been done
- What measures have been taken to make the child safe
- What have been done so far regarding the mistake;
    - ✓ *You don't need to take this issue any further if you don't wish to, as I assure you that we will be taking all the relevant steps to try to prevent this from happening again*
    - ✓ *We will fill in a critical incidence form which is an important step to ensure future consideration as regard to this issue*
    - ✓ *It will be raised and discussed in the clinical governance*
    - ✓ *All the staff are being educated*
    - ✓ *The incident is documented in the child's progress notes*
    - ✓ Suggestion for how to avoid this mistake
    - ✓ Any possible investigations for the current condition

4- **Chance for parent or child questions and concerns**
5- **Summary**

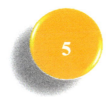

Talking to a non-compliant adolescent/parent

1- **Introduction/clarify roles, agree aims and objectives**
2- **Parent or child understanding**
3- **The main conversation bulk**

- *When were you first diagnosed?*
- *What was the impact on you and your parents and what was your reaction?*
- *Were there any complications or admission in the past few weeks?*
- *I have been asked to sit with you perhaps your control is not as it is supposed to be*
- *What do you think the reason behind this?*
- Ask about the difficulties in technique, timing, life style influence
- *Are you following any monitoring program*
- Ask about social, family and school concerns
- *Whom do you think can offer you the best support?*
- *Do you think you could benefit from educational programs, camping, activity days?*

4- **Chance for parent or child questions and concerns**
5- **Summary**

Hint;
- Don't assume that they know everything
- Show respect
- Be honest
- Thank them for being honest to you

Talking about an ethical consideration
example: disclosure of disease status

1. **Introduction/clarify roles, agree aims and objectives**
2. **Parent or child understanding**
3. **The main conversation bulk**
   - Define a question of concern
   - Advantages versus disadvantages of raising the issue
     - ✓ **Autonomy:** the patient has the right to understand his illness and to be involved in the care
     - ✓ **Beneficence:**
       - The patient will offer help if the illness is known
       - Compliance with the management
       - Reduce the child's anxiety
     - ✓ **Non-maleficence:**
       - Right to confidentiality
       - Alter self-esteem
       - Alter sensation of wellbeing
       - Protect from stigma
     - ✓ **Justice**
   - Others
     - ✓ Offer another meeting with the family or team to explain advantages and disadvantages
     - ✓ Contact specialist
     - ✓ Involve social workers and health educators
4. **Chance for parent or child questions and concerns**
5. **Summary**

Obstacles to autonomy

Parent	Ask and discuss with them their opinion
External pressure	Find it out, how to overcome
Non-understanding	Give time to understand; i.e. staged disclosure

History Taking

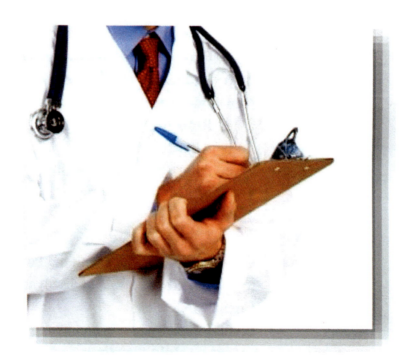

History Taking

This is not a test of your ability to take a comprehensive history, but instead it is to assess your ability to take a focused well-structured history and summarize it back addressing the main issues in concern.

Conduct of interview

1. Greet the parents and the child
2. Introduce yourself
3. Clarify the role and agree aims and objectives
4. Keep eye contact
5. Make the family at ease and make sure of their understanding
6. Be confident

History taking

1. Avoid medical phrases
2. Use open-ended and closed question as well
3. Give the parents time to speak and listen carefully to them
4. Explain the main problem to the maximum and dig deep to reach the full information
5. Explore social and family issues fully

Interpretation and management plan

1. Summarize the case in few sentences
2. Give a valid differential diagnosis and keep the rare issues to the end of your list
3. Suggest essential points in management
4. Address parent's concern fully
5. Suggest referral to other health facilities

Essential points of management (management of any medical problem)

1. **Family education:**
   - Provide them with activity programs
   - Suggest sharing in educational programs
   - Meetings with specialized health educator
   - Suggest camping days
   - Provide websites centered on parents perspectives

2. **Contact groups & organizations:**
   - Functions online through giving needed information
   - Arranges group training & group education

3. **Life style advices:**
   - Advices on sleep arrangements
   - Advices on exercise
   - Advices on diet
   - Advices on managing activities, managing time
   - Counselling bad habits; smoking, alcoholism
   - Keeping diaries

4. **Monitoring programs:**
   - Monitoring growth
   - Monitoring school
   - Monitoring specific investigation, checking blood sugar

5. **Helping with disability living allowance**
6. **Helping with special educational needs**
7. **Referral to other health facilities**
8. **Special investigations**
9. **Specific treatment**

Suggested approach for History Taking

1. **Chief complaint**
   All the primary problems in the patient's own words

2. **History of present illness**
   - Detailed history of the chief complaint
   - Chronologic order
   - Associated symptoms and relation to main complaint
   - Onset, durations, course, severity, aggravating and relieving factors and everything related to this complaint
   - Review fully the system related to the complaint; respiratory system if complaint is noisy breathing

3. **Systems review**
   General wellbeing
   Crying, irritability, poor sleeping, activity
   Skin
   Rashes, bleeding, itching, discoloration, ulceration
   EENT
   Nasal discharge, facial pain, ear discharge, hearing, vision
   Respiratory
   Runny nose, cough, wheeze, SOB, activity limitation, snoring
   Cardiac
   Infant feeding, sweating, cyanosis, chest pain, pallor, SOB
   GIT
   Appetite, diet, vomiting, pain, abdominal distention, bowel habit, stools, diarrhea, constipation, toilet training
   GU
   Pain, color, frequency, toilet training

CNS
> Headache, blurring of vision, swallowing, vomiting, convulsions, abnormal movements, steadiness, concentration, memory, attention

Musculoskeletal
> Limp / limb pain / joint swelling / pain

Pubertal
> 2ry sexual characters, menstruation

4. Past history

1. Major medical illness
2. Major surgical operations, dates, details
3. Previous admissions, reasons, duration
4. Current medication, doses, compliance, technique
5. Known allergies
6. Vaccination status in details/premature infants/high risk groups

5. Pregnancy & birth history

- **Previous abortions**
- **Pregnancy**: hypertension, diabetes, fever, bleeding, drugs
- **Gestational age** at delivery
- **Mode of delivery**
- **Neonatal**. fever, jaundice, cyanosis, respiratory support, need of O2, feeding *see page 105*

Neonatal history should be taken with extreme concentration trying to cover all the topics related to this area including diagnoses, investigations, and full management done especially if the child was premature.

6. Developmental history

Ask in general about ages of main developmental areas, gross motor, fine motor, vision, speech, hearing and social areas.

7. Nutritional history
Make it brief or if required you have to take it in details
See page 58

8. Family history
- Consanguinity
- Composition of family
- Major health problems

9. Social history
- Parent's occupation
- Second hand smoke exposure
- Living situation. house or flat, recent move
- Who cares for the child, who lives with the child
- Does anyone else help with childcare
- Pets
- School attendance, progress, bullying, friends
- Social relations

10. Others
- **Thoughts**
  What are the patients thoughts regarding their symptoms?
- **Concerns**
  Explore any worries the patient may have regarding their symptoms
- **Expectations**
  Gain an understanding of what the patient is hoping to achieve from the consultation

HINT· *You will probably finish the history taking before time, **NEVER** stay speechless, go on and ask more about social history and other parental concerns and issues, dig more in the history until you are stopped by the examiner*

Nutritional history

1. **Neonatal**
   - What was the type of feeding when born
   - When was he weaned
   - When did you introduce solid food
   - Did he need frequent feeds or overnight continuous feed

2. **Current type of feeding**
3. **Supplemental feeding program**
   Did he have any condition, which implies supplemental feeding program?

4. **Therapeutic feeding program**
   Did he have any condition, which implies therapeutic feeding program?

5. **How** is feeding given? orally, NGT, Gastrostomy
6. **Diary** Have you ever kept a food diary?

7. **Causes of failure to thrive**
   - Does he have any sort of chronic illness like heart or chest disease
   - Does he have any condition which leads to decreased oral intake
     - ✓ Inability to swallow
     - ✓ Vomiting
   - Does he have any condition which leads to decreased absorption of food

8. **GIT symptoms**
   - Nausea, vomiting
   - Abdominal colic / Abdominal distension
   - Diarrhea / Constipation

9. What is the **pattern of weight**

10. Do you think that there is any other condition responsible for his weight pattern

Reviews

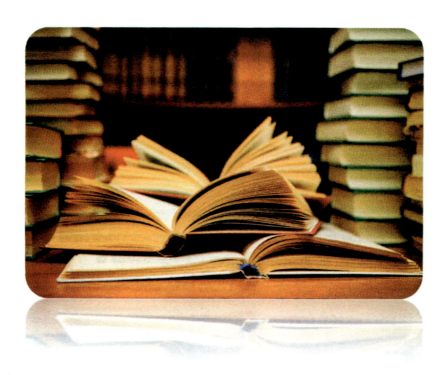

Congenital Heart Disease

8 per 1000 live-birth have CHD

Common defects:

VSD: 30%

PDA: 12%

ASD: 7%

AS, PS, COA, TOF each of   5%

Screening for CHD:

1. Family history or previous child with CHD
2. Maternal risk factors. *See below*
3. Abnormal cardiac anatomy during routine antenatal care
4. Increased nuchal translucency suggesting Down syndrome
5. Suspected one of the syndromes that are associated with CHD

Incidence is increased by:

1. Maternal SLE
2. Maternal ingestion of lithium
3. Maternal infections
4. Other anomalies or syndromes
5. Abnormal parental genotypes
6. Positive family history

Jugular venous pressure (JVP)

JVP should only be attempted in older children

Technique:

- Position the child supine on bed with head elevated 45 degree
- Turn the head slightly aside so the neck veins can be visible

Characteristics of JVP:

- It is a wave form
- Not palpable
- Rises with pressure on the liver
- Stops with pressure on the neck base
- Varies with raising or lowering the head
- Varies with respiration
- Normal value is around 4 cm above the sternal angle

Types of JVP:

a wave	right atrial contraction	increased in pulmonary hypertension

Canon a waves are seen in complete heart block

c wave	ventricular contraction	
v wave	right atrial filling	increased in tricuspid regurgitation

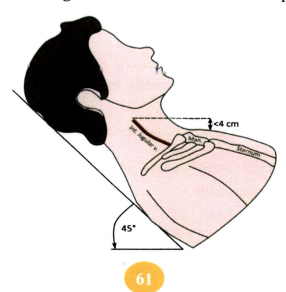

Dextrocardia

This is occurring when the heart apex points to the right

Dextrocardia can be associated with:

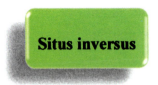 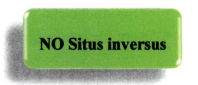

Mostly **normal** heart

- Right atria on the left
- Left atria on the right
- 3 lobed right lung on the left
- 2 lobed left lung on the right
- Stomach & spleen on the right
- Liver on the left

Mostly **abnormal** heart, may have

- Single ventricle
- VSD
- ASD
- AVSD
- Atrial transposition

- Dextrocardia is sometimes associated with asplenia or polysplenia syndrome.
- **Primary ciliary dyskinesia is**: defect in cilial structure, mobility or both. Due to ultrastructural defects in the Dynein side arms.
    - Dextrocardia
    - Bronchiectasis
    - Situs inversus
    - Infertility
    - Sinusitis
    - Chronic suppurative otitis media

Investigation. saccharin test, ciliary brush biopsy, electron microscopy

- **Kartagener syndrome** is a triad of;
    - Bronchiectasis
    - Situs inversus
    - Sinusitis

Syncope in Childhood

It is very common in childhood and mostly of a benign cause

Types:

- **Cardiogenic**: arrhythmias
- **Non-cardiogenic**: (pseudo-syncope): psychogenic
- **Neutrally mediated**.
    - Postural hypotension
    - Vaso-vagal attacks

The most important thing is taking a thorough history

Investigations:

- ECG to exclude long QT syndromes
- Exercise ECG
- Rarely EEG is needed

Management options:

- Reassurance
- Drinking good amount of water and more salt
- Fludrocortisone
- B- blocker
- Anti-arrhythmic drugs
- Implantable cardiofibrillator

Pulmonary Hypertension

Occurs when the systolic pulmonary pressure is more than 50% of systemic systolic pressure

Types:

- **Pulmonary artery Hypertension**
    - Idiopathic
    - Collagen vascular disease
    - Portal hypertension
    - Drugs, toxins
    - Persistent Pulmonary Hypertension of Newborn

- **Pulmonary venous Hypertension**
    - Left atrial/ventricular heart defects
    - Left valvular heart disease
    - External pressure on pulmonary veins

- **Pulmonary Hypertension due to respiratory disease**
    - COPD
    - Interstitial lung disease
    - Neonatal lung disease
    - High attitude

- **Pulmonary Hypertension due to thrombosis**
    - SCA
    - Pulmonary embolism

- **Pulmonary Hypertension due to direct disorder in pulmonary vasculature**
    - Sarcoidosis
    - Schistosomiasis

Persistent Pulmonary Hypertension of Newborn

Etiology:

1. Idiopathic
2. Respiratory distress syndrome
3. Congenital diaphragmatic hernia
4. B-streptococcal infection

Diagnosis:

1. Hypoxia
2. Low cardiac output
3. Loud P2
4. Oligaemic lung fields
5. Hepatomegaly
6. Echocardiographic confirmation

Management:

1. Resuscitation
2. Ventilation
3. Sedation
4. Paralysis
5. Chest physiotherapy
6. Fluid restriction
7. Medication:
    a. Nitric oxide
    b. Prostacyclin
    c. MgSO4
8. ECMO

Dilated Cardiomyopathy

Etiology:

1. Viral infection
2. Multiple blood transfusions
3. Nutritional deficiencies; selenium, thiamine
4. Family history of Autoimmune or Myopathy disease

Clinical picture:

- Exertional dyspnea, ischemia, chest pain, syncope, pulmonary edema
- Mitral regurge or Tricuspid regurge
- Signs of left or right heart failure

Investigations:

- ECG to exclude ischemia and arrhythmia
- Echocardiography
- CXR to detect arterial calcifications
- Blood work
    - CBC, serum Electrolytes, Liver function tests
    - Carnitine, Acyl-Carnitine
    - Amino acids, organic acids
    - Selenium, Thiamine levels
    - Virology; EBV, Coxaciviruses, Adenoviruses

Treatment:

- Anti-heart failure measures
- Cardiac transplant

Hypertrophic Cardiomyopathy

Risk factors:

1. History of sudden infant death syndrome
2. Infant of diabetic mother
3. Metabolic disease

Associations:

- Noonan syndrome, Fredreich's ataxia, Neurofibromatosis
- Mucopolysaccharidosis, Hypo- and hyper- thyroidism
- Cataracts, ataxia, deafness, myopathy

Investigations:

- ECG
- Echocardiography
- CXR
- Blood works
    - CBC, serum Electrolytes, Liver function tests
    - Carnitine, Acyl-Carnitine
    - Amino acids, organic acids
    - Thyroid functions
- Urine
    - Glycosaminoglycan, Organic acid, VMA

Clinical picture:

- Exertional dyspnea, ischemia, chest pain, syncope, pulmonary edema
- Mitral regurge

Treatment: B-blocker, Myectomy

Pericarditis

Etiology:

- Infection.
    - Staphylococcus
    - Tuberculosis
    - Coxaciviruses
    - Enteroviruses
- Oncologic
- Rheumatic fever
- Systemic lupus erythematosus
- Juvenile Rheumatoid Arthritis

Clinical picture:

- Fever
- Chest pain
- Muffled heart sounds
- Friction rub

Investigation:

- ECG *see page 235*
- Elevated ST segment
- Inverted T wave

Treatment:

- Anti-inflammatory drugs
- Treatment of effusion if present

Interventional Cardiac Catheters

ASD:	device occlusion
PDA.	coil, device
AS:	balloon dilatation
PS:	balloon dilatation
COA.	stent
Pulmonary atresia.	radiofrequency ablation
Arrhythmia.	radiofrequency ablation

Balloon atrial septostomy

- Under Echocardiographic control
- Done in TGA, severe cyanosis
- Via umbilical vein or femoral approach if older than 3 days

Wolf-Parkinson-White syndrome

This occurs as a result of an abnormal conductive tissue between the atria and ventricle other than the normal AV node

Presentation:

- Tachypnea
- Tachycardia
- Pallor
- Irritability
- Headache
- Syncope
- Chest pain
- Decreased activity

Diagnosis:

- CBC, Electrolytes, Liver function, thyroid function
- Echocardiography
- ECG: short PR interval – wide QRS – Delta wave *see page 234*

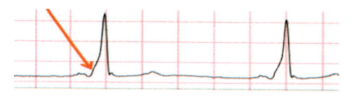

Management:

- Acute: According to the severity
    - Vagal maneuvers (Valsalva, carotid sinus massage, cold ice)
    - Adenosine
    - Synchronized DC shock
- Maintenance:
    - Amiodarone
- Definitive treatment
    - Radiofrequency ablation

Optic nerve pathway and visual defects

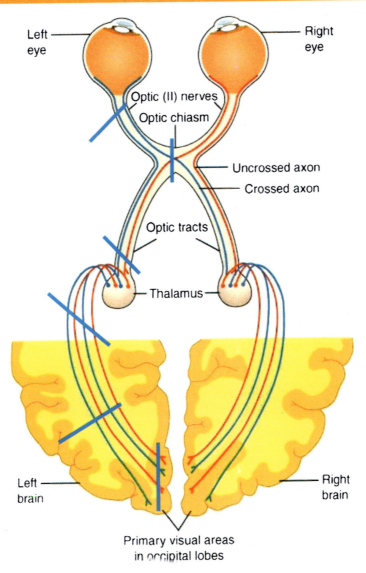

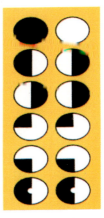

1-Blindness

2-Bitemporal hemianopia

3-Contralateral homonymous hemianopia

4-Superior quadrantopia

5-Inferior quadrantopia

6-Homonymous hemianopia with macular sparing

Ocular cranial nerve palsies

3rd Cranial nerve Oculomotor	4th Cranial nerve Trochlear	6th Cranial nerve Abducens
Diplopia	Diplopia	Diplopia
Downward and lateral gaze	Failure to downward and lateral gaze	Convergent squint
Complete ptosis		
Pupil dilatation		

Nystagmus

This is abnormal, rhythmic and involuntary eye movements with slow and fast phase

Types:

- **Cerebellar:**
    - The fast phase is directed towards the side of the lesion
- **Vestibular:**
    - The slow phase is directed towards the side of the lesion
- **Vertical:**
    - Lesions in the brain stem, may be due to phenytoin and carbamazepine
- **Ocular:**
    - Slow searching movement in blindness
- **Congenital:**
    - Bilateral, horizontal, idiopathic and improves with age

Squints

Types:

- Latent, manifest
- Alternating, monocular
- Convergent, divergent
- Non-paralytic
    - Cataract
    - Refractive errors
    - ROP
    - Retinoblastoma
- Paralytic
    - Cranial nerve defects
    - Muscle disease
    - Infections

Assessment:

1. Ocular movement
2. Corneal reflexes
3. Cover and uncover test *see next page.*

Management:

- Treatment of the cause
- Achieve best ocular alignment
- Surgery may be considered

Cover and uncover test

Cover Test

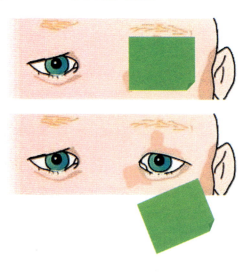

Cover one eye
look at the other eye

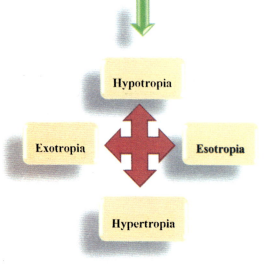

Eye ball movement

Cover / Uncover Test

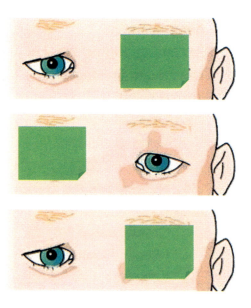

Cover one eye
then cover the other
look at the uncovered

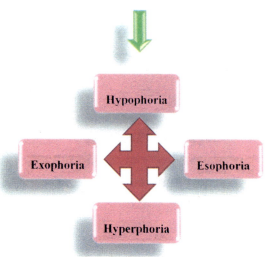

Eye ball movement

Weber and Rinne Test

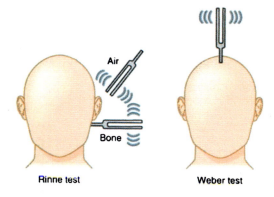

BC: Bone conduction

AC. Air conduction

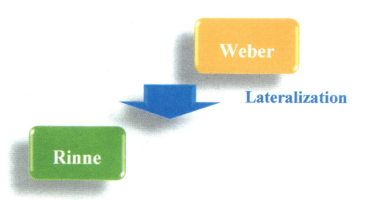

| BC > AC = conductive hearing loss | BC > AC = combined |
| AC > BC = normal | AC > BC = sensorineural |

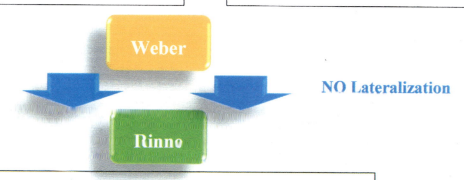

Both BC > AC   =   Bilateral conductive

Both AC > BC   =   normal

Audiometry / Audiogram

- Performed for ages more than 4 years
- Both ears are examined separately
- It delivers sounds at different frequencies

Audiogram:

X	axis frequencies in Hertz
Y	axis hearing level in Decibel
O	Air conduction (AC) right ear
X	Air conduction (AC) left ear
Δ	Bone conduction (unmasked)
[	Bone conduction (BC) in right ear masked
]	Bone conduction (BC) in left ear masked

Air conduction: assesses all auditory system
Bone conduction: assesses from cochlea and beyond

- **Conductive loss:** difference between AC, BC
- **Sensorineural loss:** equal impairment
- **Mixed:** AC>BC

Normal Audiogram

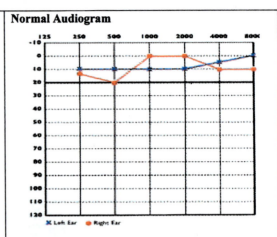

Conductive hearing loss

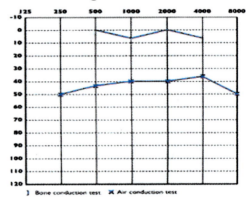

Mixed hearing loss

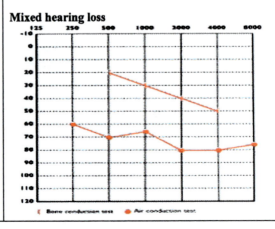

Normal values

Normal	-10-20
Mild to moderate	20-40
Severe	60-80
Profound	90-120

Causes of Global developmental delay

Pre-natal
- Chromosomal abnormalities
- Congenital infection
- Teratogens
- Brain malformation

Natal
- Prematurity
- Hypoxic ischemic encephalopathy
- Infection
- Trauma
- Kernicterus

Post-natal
- Trauma
- Infection
- Intracranial hemorrhage

Metabolic
- Aminoaciduria
- Mucopolysaccharidosis
- Galactosemia
- Gaucher disease
- Niemann-Pick Disease

Endocrine
- Hypothyroidism

Tests for Visual acuity

Newborn	:	Examine both eyes
6 weeks	:	Examine, fix & follow 90°
12 weeks	:	Examine, fix & follow 180°
10 months	:	Pick-up raisin
3 years	:	Preferential looking tests
3 years	:	Gardner tests
4 years	:	Snellen chart

Tests for Hearing acuity

Newborn:
1. Oto-acoustic emission. Probe in ear (cochlea should be normal)
2. Auditory Brainstem Response: scalp electrodes

8 months:

Distraction tests

Distractor

Baby

Sound

2 years:

- Performance test
- Speech discrimination
- Visual Reinforcement Audiometry

4 years:

Pure tone audiometry

Pseudobulbar Palsy

- Upper motor neuron lesion of lower cranial nerves
- Associated with Cerebral Palsy

Signs:
- Dry voice
- Stiff tongue
- Exaggerated jaw reflex
- Preserved gag plus palatal reflex

Facial Palsy

- Examine skin. erythema migrans
- Examine ears: vesicles

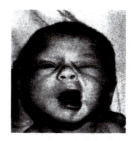

Causes:

LMNL	UMNL
<ul><li>Congenital</li><li>Traumatic</li><li>Inflammatory</li><li>Infection:<ul><li>Viral</li><li>Ramsey Hunt syndrome</li><li>Lyme syndrome</li><li>Otitis media</li></ul></li><li>Intracranial tumor</li><li>Bell's palsy</li></ul>	<ul><li>Cerebral Palsy</li><li>Mobius syndrome</li><li>Trauma</li></ul>

Ptosis

Causes:

Syndromic	Neurologic
<ul><li>Noonan</li><li>Rubenstein Taybi syndrome</li><li>Marcus Gun</li><li>Smith-Lemli-Opitz</li></ul>	<ul><li>Horner</li><li>3rd nerve palsy</li><li>Myasthenia Gravis</li><li>Myotonic dystrophy</li><li>Neuroblastoma</li><li>Rhabdomyosarcoma</li><li>Congenital</li></ul>

Myasthenia Gravis

- Progressive weakness (proximal) associated with ocular problems, ptosis.
- Decreased acetylcholine transferase within Neuro-muscular Junction.

Investigations
1. Anti-acetylcholine receptor antibodies
2. Anticholinesterase test
3. EMG
4. Muscle biopsy
5. CT/MRI

Treatment
- Anticholinesterase (Pyridostigmine)
- Immunosuppression (steroids, azathioprine, cyclosporine)
- IVIG
- Plasmapheresis
- Thymectomy

Autistic Spectrum Disorder

Defects:

- **Social**
    - Failure to develop relationships
    - Emotional disorder
- **Communication:**
    - Delay in spoken language
    - Failure to start conversations
    - Failure to communicate with others
    - Lack of eye contact
- **Repetitive & stereotype behavior:**
    - Adherence to routine
    - Lack of imaginative play
    - Repetitive motor manners
- **Other associations:**
    - Intellectual impairment 50%
    - Epilepsy 30%
    - Hearing, visual disorders
    - Dyspraxia

Management: *see page 54*

1. Family education
2. Contact groups & organizations
3. Life style advices
4. Monitoring programs
5. Helping with disability living allowance
6. Helping with special educational needs
7. Referral to other health facilities

Dyspraxia

Difficulty performing coordinated actions

- **Young child:**
    - Slow gross motor development
    - Poor motor skills
    - Difficulty in dressing
    - Difficulty in pencil grip

- **Older child:**
    - Slow school progress
    - Reduced attention
    - Poor writing
    - Poor reading
    - Difficulty in math

Assessment BY:

- Pediatrician
- Occupational therapist
- Speech and language assessment

Management: *see page 54*

1. Family education
2. Contact groups & organizations
3. Life style advices
4. Monitoring programs
5. Helping with disability living allowance
6. Helping with special educational needs
7. Referral to other health facilities

ADHD

- 1% of school age children
- More common in boys

Triad of:

1. Inattention
2. Hyperactivity
3. Impulsiveness

In association with:

1. Persisting features more than 6 months
2. Occurs in more than one setting
3. Social and academic impairment
4. No other explanation

Management: *see page 54*

1. Family education
2. Contact groups & organizations
3. Life style advices
4. Monitoring programs
5. Helping with disability living allowance
6. Helping with special educational needs
7. Referral to other health facilities

Plus

Methylphenidate

- Not recommended under 6 years of age
- To be taken twice daily (morning, lunch)
- Monitor height weight, pulse, BP
- Causes hypertension, growth retardation
- Drug holiday is recommended yearly
- Drug should be stopped if ineffective

Bullying

When one child abuses power to cause pain or distress to other child in repeated occasions

Bullies	Victim
- Emotional disorder - Conduct disorder - Social disorder	- Anxiety - Unsecure - Low self-esteem - Headache - Abdominal pain - Bed wetting

School refusal

Risk factors	Characteristics
- Separation anxiety - Specific phobia - Depression - Bullying	- Good academic achievement - Home oppositional - School conformist

Functional abdominal pain

1. Common, 10% in school age children
2. Girls > boys
3. > 5 years of age
4. Family history
5. Mostly non-organic

Categories:
1. Function dyspepsia — post feeds
2. Irritable bowel — loose stools alternating constipation
3. Abdominal migraines — pallor, nausea, vomiting and headache
4. Functional abdominal pain syndrome (by exclusion)

Factors Suggest Organic Pain:
1. Age < 5 years
2. Family history of Inflammatory Bowel Disease
3. Constitutional manifestation. fever, weight loss
4. Vomiting "Bilious"
5. Bloody stool
6. Pain away from umbilicus or referred pain
7. Pain that awakens the child at night
8. Urinary symptoms
9. Perianal disease

Associations:
Nervous Personality   -   Perfectionist   -   School Absence

Management: *"Pain is real"*

- Reassurance
- Education
- Life style (exercise, school)
- Diet control
- Diary of Symptoms

Vaccination schedule

Date	Vaccine	
Neonate	BCG (high risk)	
2 months	DTaP-IPV-HiB	Pneumococcal vaccine
3 months	DTaP-IPV-HiB	Meningococcal C vaccine
4 months	DTaP-IPV-HiB	Pneumococcal vaccine
		Meningococcal C vaccine
12 months	HiB	Meningococcal C vaccine
13 months	MMR	Pneumococcal vaccine
3.5 years	MMR	
	DTaP-IPV	
10-13 years	BCG	
13-18 years	DT-IPV	

Contraindication to vaccinations	Contraindication to Live vaccines

▪ Acute illness
▪ Local reaction (extensive redness, swelling)
▪ General reaction (fever, anaphylaxis, bronchospasm, collapse)
	▪ Steroids
	  o 1 mg/kg/day for 1 month
	  o 2 mg/kg/day for 1 week
	▪ Chemotherapy in the last 6 months
	▪ BMT in the last 6 months
	▪ IVIG in the last 3 months
	▪ Impaired cell mediated immunity

HIV should not receive: **BCG, oral typhoid vaccine, yellow fever vaccine**

MMR should not be given to those with **neomycin/kanamycin** allergy
- No link between MMR and autism
- No link between MMR and inflammatory bowel disease
- Separate vaccine is harmful

Capillary Hemangioma

- Appears first few weeks of life
- Common in preterm

Phases:

1. Proliferative
2. Stabilization
3. Regression. 50% in 5 years, 90% in 9 years

Complications:

- Ulceration
- Bleeding
- Infection
- Heart failure

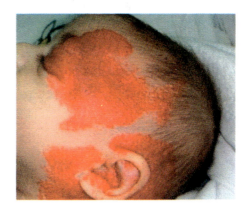

Kasabach Merrit:

Hemangioma + thrombocytopenia + micoangiopathic hemolytic anemia

Management:

- Propranolol
- Excision
- Laser
- Alpha interferon
- Steroids

Port-Wine Stain

- Capillary malformation
- Persists throughout life
- Associated with Sturge Weber, Klippel Trennuary Weber syndrome

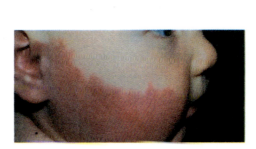

Atopic Eczema

1. 10-20% of children
2. 70% have positive family history
3. Common in first 6 months of life
4. Common in face, scalp and flexures
5. 2ry infection by: staphylococcus, streptococcus, herpes
6. Resolve in 50% at age of 6 years, and 90% at age of 14 years

Risk factors:

- Allergens: nickle, chrome
- Irritants: chemical, wool
- Infections
- Environmental: mites, pets
- Dry skin
- Emotional stress
- Heat, sweeting

Differential diagnosis: seborrheic dermatitis, jobs' syndrome, WAS, contact dermatitis

Management:

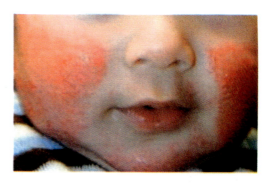

1. Emollients
2. Steroid cream
3. Zinc impregnated bandages
4. Wet wraps
5. Tacrolimus
6. Antihistaminics
7. Antibiotics
8. Acyclovir
9. Systemic steroids

Psoriasis

1. Common at 5-9 years in girls, 15-19 years in boys
2. 10% 1st degree, 50% both parents, 70% monozygotic twins
3. Common at extensors
4. Increased epidermal turnover
5. Characterized by relapsing and remissions
6. Nail involvement: pits, onycholysis
7. Arthropathy with HLA B27

Types: common, guttate, erythrodermic, pustular

Risk factors:

- Trauma
- Infection
- Sunlight
- Hypocalcemia
- Puberty
- Stress
- HIV

Management:

1. Emollients
2. Tar based emollients
3. Steroid cream
4. Vitamin D derivative cream
5. Dithranol preparations
6. UVB phototherapy
7. Systemic: methotrexate, cyclosporine

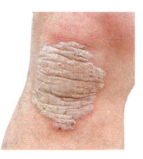
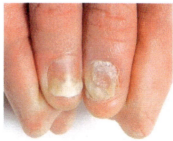

Basics of Cardiac Arrest

1. Approach. **SAFE** Technique

    Shout for help

    Approach with care

    Free from danger

    Evaluate

2. Airway opening:
    - Head tilt, Chin lift
    - Jaw Thrusts

3. Breathing:

    Look   chest movements
    Listen breath sounds
    Feel   breath warmth

4. Rescue breathing: 5 times

5. Check circulation

6. Chest compression.   Rate of 100/min
    - Infants/child   15:2
    - After puberty   30:2

chain of survival

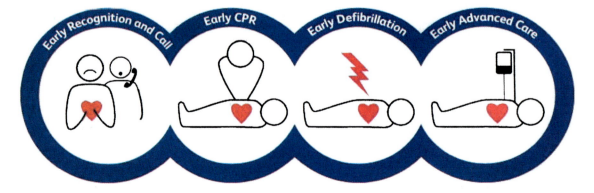

Withdrawal of life sustaining medical treatment

Professional guidance

5 Situation when it is ethical to do so:

1) Brain dead Child:

Criteria of Brain Stem Death agreed by 2 Practitioners.

2) Permanent Vegetative State:

Reliant on others for all care with no reaction or relation to outside world.

3) No chance Situation:

Severe disease, and treatment delays death with no alleviation of suffering.

4) No Purpose:

Survive with treatment but degree of physical, mental impairment is great.

5) Unbearable:

Family & child feel further treatment unbearable in progressive illness.

Decisions should be made by the team with no rush & all evidence available.

Withdrawal should be associated with:
- Palliative, terminal care needs, Symptoms alleviation.
- Maintaining human dignity and comfort.

When offering withdrawal, you should explain that: ## Ethical guidance

1. He has awful life.
2. He has serious damages & disabilities.
3. His body can't fight anymore.
4. None of the treatment option come out with positive results.
5. Treatment prolongs his suffering.
6. Death is imminent & irreversibly close.

Confidentiality

"No disclosure without consent"

Justification:

1. Respect of Autonomy
2. Beneficence.
3. Non-maleficence.
4. Justice.
5. Confidentiality is Professional.
6. Duty of virtuous Doctor is to keep things confidential.

Principles:

1. No disclosure without consent.
2. Necessary information should only be disclosed.
3. Data made anonymous if serves the purpose.
4. Disclose within health care team if no specific objection.

Disclosure is legal when:

1. Birth and Death.
2. Infectious disease.
3. Request from the court.

Disclosure is discretionary when:

1. Harm to 3rd party
2. Investigating a crime; child abuse

Contraception in teens

Ethical Justification:

1. Respect of Autonomy
2. Beneficence.
3. Non-maleficence.
4. Justice (right to health, information, identity).

Legal Justification:

1. Aware & understand implication to self & family
2. Persistence refusal to inform parents.
3. She will continue to do so regardless advice.
4. Health will suffer if not prescribed.
5. Contraception is in her best interest.

Abortion

Legal if not exceeding 24 months when.

1. Physical or mental harm to mother
2. Physical or mental harm to child.
3. Continuation for mother carries more risk than if terminated.

Audit

- This is an examination or review which establishes to what extent a performance or a condition conforms to criteria & standards of practice.
- Best way to improve patient care by comparing what is done to what should be done.
- Examples. Guidelines

Audit cycle:
1. Identify a topic
2. Set the standards & criteria that should be definable, measurable and of good evidence
3. Measure current practice against standards
4. Identify key priorities for change
5. Implement changes
6. Re-audit to see what difference has been made

Types of clinical studies

Treatment Studies:
- Randomized clinical studies
    - Blind
    - Double blind
    - Non-blind

Observational Studies:
- Cohort
    - Prospective
    - Retrospective
- Case Control
- Cross sectional

Evidence based medicine

Definition:

The conscientious, explicit & judicious use of current best evidence to make management decisions for patient.

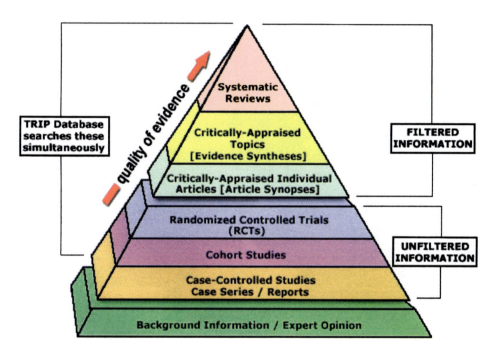

Stages:

1. Faced with a clinical problem
2. Define a question
3. Search for latest evidence
4. Is it applicable for the patient
5. Consider the
    i. Evidence
    ii. Clinical experience
    iii. Patient preferences
6. Evaluate all the above & formulate care plan.

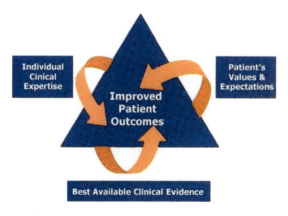

Clinical Governance – *control and direct with authority*

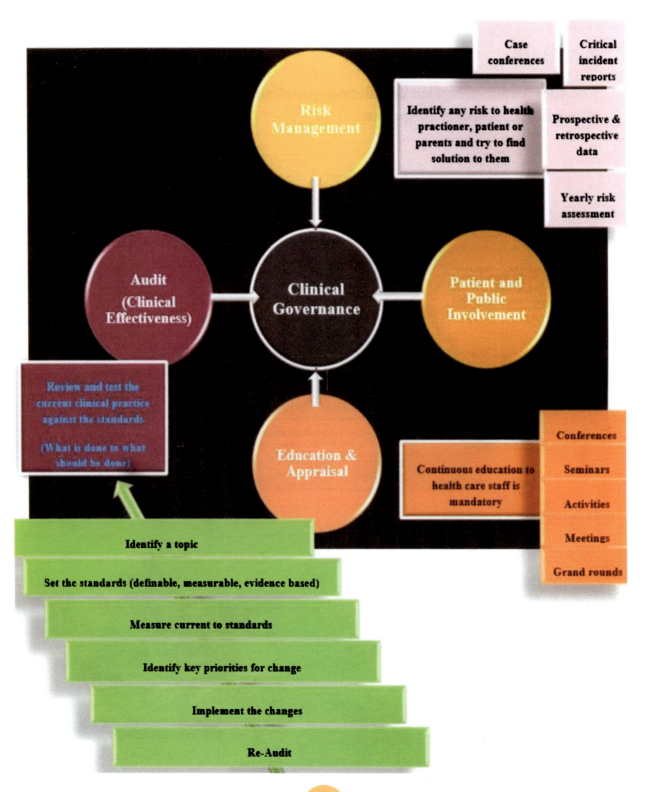

Inheritance of Down syndrome

3 Types of inheritance

1) Non-disjunction: 94%

Failure of division of chromosome 21 during meiosis.

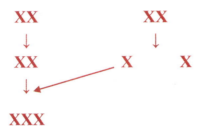

2) Translocation: 5%

Part of one chromosome (15, 22, and 21) is attached to Chromosome 21

3) Mosaicism: 1%

Some cells have 3 copies of Chromosome 21, others are normal due to abnormal mitosis post fertilization.

- Inheritance increased with age, especially mothers > 35 years
- If mother has one child with Down syndrome, chance to have another child is 1:100.
- Mother of translocation has recurrence of 15%.
- Father of translocation has recurrence of 2.5%

Screening tests

Screening aims to prevent avoidable morbidity and mortality of a disease

Requirements:

1. Important health problem
2. Available test for diagnosis
3. Acceptable treatment
4. Early treatment improves prognosis
5. Latent or asymptomatic disease
6. Economic

Current screening program at birth include:

- Congenital hypothyroidism
- Phenylketonuria
- SCA thalassemia
- MCADD
- Cystic fibrosis
- +/- Galactosemia
- +/- Duchenne muscular dystrophy

Screening Tests:

Formula	Term	Description
a / a+c	**Sensitivity**	proportion of true +ve identified by test
d / b+d	**Specificity**	proportion of true –ve identified by test
a / a+b	**+ve predictive value**	proportion of those test +ve & diseased
d / c+d	**- ve predictive value**	proportion of those test –ve & not diseased

	diseased	non-diseased
+ve	a	b
-ve	c	d

Screening for Down syndrome

Several tests are used to screen for Down syndrome during the antenatal period

It includes:

- **Combined test:**

  Week 11-13
  - Ultrasound — Nuchal translucency
  - Blood test — β-HCG – Pregnancy associated plasma proteins (PAPP)

- **Quadruple test:**

  Week 15-20
  - Blood test — Alpha fetoprotein – β-HCG – PAPP – Inhibin A

- **Definitive test:**

  To detect chromosomal abnormalities

  - Week 15 — Amniocentesis
  - Week 9-14 — Chorionic villous sampling
  - Week 18 — PUBS

Genomic imprinting

Every character is expressed by genes from both parents, however some characters are expressed only by paternal or maternal gene.

Syndromes will be the result of:

- Deletion of paternal or maternal chromosome or
- Uniparental disomy (both copies of chromosomes derived from one parent)

Examples:

1. Prader Willi
   - Deletion of paternal chromosome 15
   - Uniparental disomy (maternal)

2. Angelman
   - Deletion of Maternal Chromosome 15
   - Uniparental disomy (paternal)

3. Russel-silver
   - Deletion on Chromosome 7

4. Beckwith Weidmann
   - Deletion on Chromosome 11

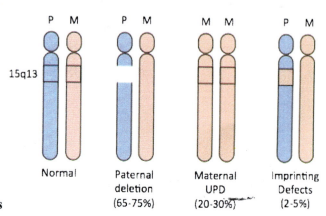

Prader Willi genetics

DiGeorge syndrome

- Also called **velo-cardio-facial** syndrome
- It's an immunodeficiency syndrome results from abnormal development of the 3rd and 4th pharyngeal arches
- Triad of hypocalcemia, CHD, immune defects
- Genetic abnormality in form of deletion of 22q detected by FISH

Characteristics:

- Low-set ears
- Hypertelorism
- Cleft lip +/- palate
- Micrognathia

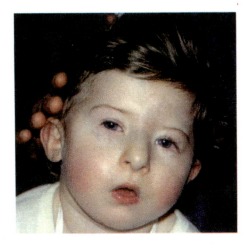

Immune defect result from absent thymus and cell mediated immunodeficiency

Management:

- Treatment of CHD
- Aggressive treatment of infections
- Bone marrow transplantation

Breast Feeding Promotion

There are 10 steps for proper breast feeding promotion:

1. Written policy of breastfeeding & communicate between health care staff

2. Train them to implement this policy

3. Educate mothers about benefits of breastfeed.

4. Start half hour after delivery

5. Show how to breast feed & maintain lactation.

6. No drinks, no food.

7. No teats, no pacifiers.

8. Breastfeed on demand.

9. Allow roaming in, 24hr/day together with the baby

10. Foster establishment of breastfeeding support group after discharge from hospital.

Infant feeding

Breast Milk

Amount/100ml	Contents	Daily Requirements per kg
70 kcal	Calories	110-120 kcal
7.5gm	CHO	3.5 – 11gm
1.1gm	Proteins	3-3.5 gm
4.2gm	Fat	20% of calories
	Na	2-3 mmol
	K	2-3 mmol
	Ca	2-3 mmol

Advantages of breast milk:

1. ↓ Respiratory and gastrointestinal infection
2. ↓ Necrotizing Enterocolitis
3. ↓ Infantile Colic
4. ↓ Diabetes
5. ↓ Atopic eczema
6. ↑ Neurologic development
7. ↑ Immunity

Food Supplements:

- **CHO** — Caloreen, Maxiguel
- **Fat** — Calogen, liquigen (MCT)
- **Combined** — Duocal
- **Protein** — whole protein, peptides, amino acids

Normal milk 13% → 65 kcal, 1.5 gm protein

Concentrated milk 15% → 75 kcal, 1.7 gm protein /100ml

Umbilical artery catheterization

- Common NICU Procedure
- Usually during 5-7 days of birth & rare 7-10 days

Indications:

1. Continuous BP monitoring
2. Blood Sampling
3. ABG Sampling
4. Exchange Transfusion
5. Maintenance Fluids
6. Angiography

Contraindications:

- Omphalocele
- Omphalitis
- Peritonitis
- NEC

Anesthesia:

Not indicated because there are no nerve fibers in the umbilical cord.

If struggling neonate → sedation with midazolam

Complications:

1. Mal-positioning, vessel perforation, peritoneal perforation
2. Thrombosis, embolism, vasospasm
3. Bleeding, infection, NEC
4. Intestinal necrosis, perforation

Preterm babies

It is defined as birth before 37 week gestation

- **Risk factors:**
    - Age <20, >40
    - Low socioeconomic status
    - Premature rapture of membranes
    - Poor nutrition
    - Anemia
    - Smoking
    - Infection
    - Uterine and cervical abnormalities

- **Outcome:**

    Survival

22 weeks	1%
23 weeks	10%
24 weeks	25%
25 weeks	45%

    Neurodevelopmental disabilities at 30 weeks or more

No	49%
Severe	23%
Moderate	25%
died	2%
Lost follow up	1%

Preterm problems:

Respiratory	Cardiac	GIT	CNS	Genitourinary	Others
Surfactant deficiency Chronic lung disease Meconium aspiration Pneumonia	PDA Hypotension Cyanosis	NEC	IVH PVL Seizures ROP HIE	Hematuria Acute renal failure	Decreased hearing due to use of aminoglycosides, IVH, Jaundice Decreased vision due to ROP, PVL

Hemolytic disease of Newborn

- Very serious bleeding disorder
- Timing:
    - Early   2-4 hours at birth
    - Classic   1-2 weeks after birth
    - Late   4-6 weeks after birth

Risk factors:

- Prematurity
- Breast feeding
- Liver Disease
- Maternal Anticonvulsant therapy
- Traumatic delivery

Vitamin K is not found in many foods & not in breast milk

Management:

Prophylaxis: Vitamin K

Orally   **IM**

- Some studies showed that Oral route is less effective than IM
- Other studies recommend IM for High risk Patients and Oral form in Low risk Patients
- Taken at birth, 1 week and 4 weeks
- **No** relation with Cancer has been documented

Intraventricular hemorrhage

Germinal matrix is rich in capillary network which is very delicate and can easily be affected by the change is cerebral blood flow

Risk factors:

- **P**rematurity
- **P**DA
- **P**neumothorax
- **P**erinatal asphyxia
- Hypercapnia, Metabolic acidosis, Hypotension

Timing:

- First 24 hours   50%
- First week   50%

Stages:

[1] Germinal matrix bleeding
[2] IVH with no dilatation
[3] IVH with dilatation
[4] Parenchymal and peri-ventricular leukomalacia

Presentation:

- Stage 1 & 2   incidental on scan
- Stage 3   shock
- Stage 4   shock + seizures + hypotonia

Cerebral palsy and neurodevelopmental delay occurs in:

- 4%   stage 1 and 2
- 50%   stage 2 plus dilatation and stage 3
- 75%   any lesion requiring a shunt surgery
- 90%   stage 4

Other complication include: post hemorrhagic ventricular dilatation, PVL

Necrotizing enterocolitis

It is a condition that mainly affects preterm infants

Pathology: Triad of

1. Hypoxic-ischemic bowel injury
2. Bacterial colonization
3. Enteral feeding

Nitric oxide is produced in large amounts which may lead to apoptosis

Risk factors:

- Premature rupture of membranes
- PDA
- Perinatal asphyxia
- Prematurity
- Polycythemia
- Umbilical catheterization
- Low birth weight

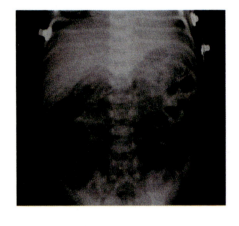

Presentation:

- Stage I. temperature instability – lethargy   vomiting – abdominal distension
- Stage II. upper & lower GI bleeding   pneumatosis intestinalis
- Stage III. sepsis – shock

X-Ray: air around liver – football sign (central abdominal lucency) – Wrigler sign (visualize both sides of bowel) – scrotal gas

Complication:

Perforation – sepsis – DIC   short bowel syndrome – stricture   recurrence

Treatment:

NPO – NGT – TPN – IV fluids   IV antibiotics

Surgery in complicated cases: laparotomy, resection of the bowel, colostomy

Developmental Dysplasia of the Hip

Risk factors:

- First baby
- Female
- Family history
- Breech presentation
- Oligohydramnios
- Torticollis
- Talipes

Types of affection:

Dislocated   **Dislocatable**   **unstable**

Test: should be done as regular screening test for each newborn

Ultrasound is not done as a regular screening tool in every hospital

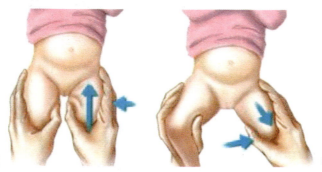

Barlow test   **Ortolani test**

Treatment:

- Orthopedic referral
- Follow up for unstable joint
- Pavlik's harness for dislocated and dislocatable joints

Complication of Pavlik's harness

- Failure
- Avascular necrosis of head of femur
- Interference with bonding

Erb's Palsy

This is a brachial plexus injury affecting C5, C6

Risk factors:

- Difficult labour
- Large birth weight
- Forceps or vacuum extraction
- Shoulder dystocia
- Family history
- Multiparity

Clinical picture:

- Adducted arm
- Internal rotation at shoulder
- Extended elbow
- Flexed wrist

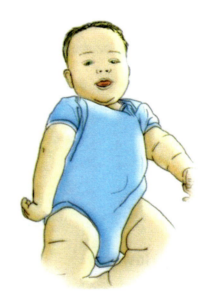

MRI is the standard and best to diagnose

Management:

- Physiotherapy
- Occupational therapy

Gastrostomy

Indication:

- Inability to move the food from the mouth to the stomach
    - Neurologic
    - Inability to swallow
    - Obstruction
- Gut decompression

Technique:

- Supine position and head is 30 degree elevated
- 4 hours fasting prior to the procedure
- Sedation or more agents like ketamine can be used if child is annoyed

Complications:

- Complication of anesthesia
- Aspiration
- Bleeding
- Infection
- Perforation of intestine
- Leakage
- Fistula
- Ulceration
- Pain

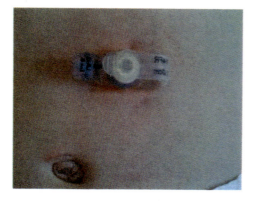
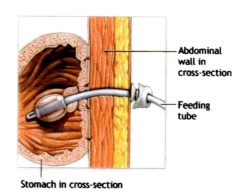

Acrodermatitis enterropathica

- It is an autosomal recessive disorder
- Due to impaired zinc absorption in the gut

Presentation:

- Peri-oral and perianal rash
- Chronic diarrhea
- Repeated Infection
- Reddish tent hair
- Candida Infection

Investigation:

- Serum zinc
- White cell zinc level
- Metallothionein level

Management:

- Oral zinc

Abetalipoproteinemia

- It is an autosomal recessive disorder
- Failure of chylomicron formation, impaired absorption of long chain fatty acid

Presentation:

- Malabsorption
- Abdominal distension
- Foul smelling, bulky stool
- Neuropathy, ataxia, retinitis pigmentosa

Investigation:

- ↓ Cholesterol
- ↓ Triglyceride
- Acanthocytes in peripheral blood film

Management:

MCT
Vitamin A, D, E, K

Cow's milk protein intolerance

Clinical Spectrum:

1. Type I hypersensitivity
2. Delayed hypersensitivity
3. Enteropathy
4. Allergic colitis
5. Non-specific: colic, constipation, chestiness, URTI

Diagnosis:

- Goldman Criteria. Symptoms disappear when antigen is removed
- Skin Prick Test, RAST

Management:

- Milk substitute with hydrolyzed protein
- Adrenaline pen if there is history of anaphylaxis

Peanut Allergy:

- Clinical picture varies from simple rash and urticarial to anaphylaxis
- Child with early onset of allergy will grow out fit
- Diagnosis is by skin prick test
- Adrenaline pen should be kept always ready

Gastroesophageal reflux

- Passage of Gastric Content to lower esophagus

Presentation:

Typical	Atypical (chest)
1. Regurgitation	1. Wheezes
2. Nausea, vomiting	2. Cough
3. Epigastric discomfort	3. Stridor
4. Dysphagia	4. Cyanosis
5. Hiccups	5. Apnea

Investigations:

- PH study (Gold standard)
    - Number of episodes
    - Number of episodes > 5 minutes
    - Duration
    - % of time PH < 4
- Upper GI endoscope, biopsy

Management:

- Reassurance, lifestyle, feeding posture, large volume food
- Avoid tea, coffee, and chocolate

1. H2 blocker, antacids
2. Proton pump inhibitors (Omeprazole)
3. Prokinetics (metoclopramide, domperidone)
4. Surgery if medical treatment fails

Intussusception

- Invagination of one portion of the intestine into another
- Peak incidence is between 6-9 months
- Mostly ileocecal

Caused by:

- Meckel's diverticulum
- Intestinal Polyps
- Lymphoma
- Henoch schonlein purpura

Presentation:

- Abdominal pain
- Vomiting (bile stained)
- Perioral pallor
- Irritability
- Blood Stained Stools
- Abdominal mass

Diagnosis:

- Plan abdominal X-ray
- Abdomen US

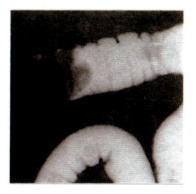

Treatment:

- Air enema reduction
- Surgery if conservative measures fail

Metabolic disorders

Clues in History:

1. Consanguineous parents
2. History of SIDS
3. Previous abortions
4. Maternal illness during pregnancy
5. History of encephalopathic or tachypneic attacks
6. Timing:
   - Neonatal period
   - Weaning
   - Infections
   - Puberty
7. Symptom free before introduction of food

Examination:

- Dysmorphic features
- Eye examination
- Organomegaly

Investigations:

1. Blood gases
2. Glucose
3. Lactate
4. Ammonia
5. Amino acids
6. Organic acid
7. Ketones
8. Acylcarnitine

Acid base status

Metabolic acidosis: ↓ PH ↓ CO2 ↓HCO3

↑ Acid Load.
- Diabetic ketoacidosis
- Lactic acidosis
- Organic acidosis
- Salicylate poisoning

↓ Acid Excretion:
- Renal tubular acidosis
- Renal failure

↑ Bicarbonate loss.
- Diarrhea
- Villous atrophy

Metabolic Alkalosis: ↑ PH ↑CO2 ↑HCO3

↑ Acid loss.
- Chloride losing diarrhea
- Pyloric stenosis
- Cushing
- Cystic fibrosis
- Bartter syndrome

Respiratory acidosis: ↓ PH ↑CO2 ↑HCO3

CO2 retention.
- Encephalopathy
- Kyphoscoliosis
- Pleural effusion, Pneumothorax
- Airway obstruction

Respiratory Alkalosis: ↑ PH ↓ CO2 ↓HCO3

- Hyperammonemia
- Salicylate poisoning

Galactosemia

- Autosomal recessive disorder
- Galactose 1 phosphate uridyl-transferase deficiency
- Increased toxic effect of galactose 1 phosphate

Presentation:

Neonatal.
- Jaundice, Organomegaly
- Cataract, coagulopathy
- E-coli, sepsis

Later   Growth failure, rickets

Investigation:

- Enzymology
- Reducing substance in urine

Management:

Strict galactose/lactose free diet

Maternal conditions affecting newborn

Diabetes:
- ↑ risk of congenital heart disease, hypertrophic cardiomyopathy
- Sacral agenesis, neural tube defect
- Hypoglycemia, ↓ Ca, ↓Mg

Hypertension:
- SGA, neutropenia, thrombocytopenia

Maternal Thyroid Disease:
- Neonatal Thyrotoxicosis.
    - ✓ transient
    - ✓ transplacental thyroid stimulating Antibodies

Systemic lupus erythematosus (SLE)
- Congenital complete heart block
- Butterfly rash
- Small for gestational age

Myasthenia Gravis:
- Transient neonatal myasthenia gravis

Thrombocytopenia:
- Neonatal iso-immune thrombocytopenia (mother with ITP)
- Neonatal Allo-immune thrombocytopenia (mother with no Human Platelets Antigen 1a - HPA1a)

Alcohol:
- Small for gestational age, microcephaly, CHD, mid-facial hypoplasia, thin lip

Opiates:
- Withdrawal symptoms

ECMO

It is a machine used when there is a membrane which allow the lung to recover from respiratory failure.

Indication:

1. Persistent pulmonary hypertension of the newborn
2. Meconium aspiration syndrome, RDS
3. Congenital diaphragmatic hernia

Pre-requisites:

1. Reversible lung disease
2. Weight > 2kg
3. > 35 weeks gestational
4. Oxygenation index > 40
5. Cranial US No ICH
6. No clotting abnormalities

Types:

- Veno-arterial
- Veno-venous

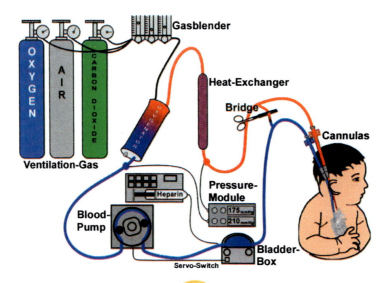

Esophageal atresia (EA) / trachea-esophageal fistula (TEF)

Types:
- Blind proximal esophagus, distal TEF 87%
- Esophageal atresia, no fistula 8%
- Proximal ± distal fistula

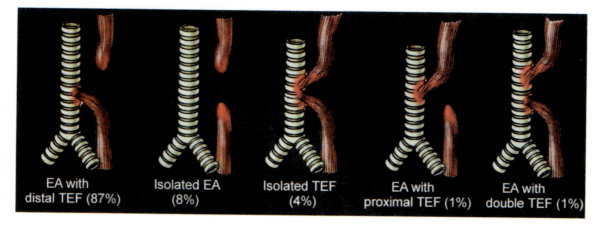

Presentation:
- Polyhydramnios
- Excessive salivation
- Respiratory Distress, choking, cyanosis
- Abdominal distension, vomiting
- Inability to pass NGT

CXR: absent gas in gut if no fistula

Management:
- Respiratory support
- Replogle tube for continuous suction
- Surgery: division of fistula, end to end esophageal anastomosis

Do not forget to do: Echo, spinal US, Karyotyping, renal US

To exclude associated conditions; i.e. VATER, VACTERL

Neonatal seizures

- 100/100,000 neonates per year

Types:
- Toxic
- Clonic
- Myoclonic

Etiology:
1. HIE, ICH
2. Intracranial infections
3. Metabolic disorders (MSUD, OA, UCD)
4. Electrolyte disorder (↓glucose, ↓Ca, ↓Mg)
5. Malformation syndrome
6. Benign Neonatal seizures

Important Parts in history:
- Family history (syndromes, neonatal convulsions)
- Pregnancy history (TORCH)
- Delivery history (Trauma, HIE)
- Postnatal history (fever, infection, trauma)

Investigation:
- Cranial US, CT, MRI Brain
- EEG
- Ca, Mg, glucose
- TORCH screening
- Metabolic screening
- CSF examination

Management:
- Phenobarbitone, if no response → phenytoin
- Maintain for 3-6 months, determine the duration by EEG
- Tapering when attempting to stop

Neonatal hypoglycemia

Blood glucose ≤ 2.6 mmol/L

Causes:

↑ Demand:
- Infection
- Asphyxia
- IUGR
- Preterm
- Hypothermia

Hyperinsulinism:
- Infant of diabetic mother
- Adenoma of the islet cells
- Beckwith Weidemann syndrome

Endocrinal:
- Growth hormone deficiency
- Congenital adrenal hyperplasia

Metabolic:
- GSD, Galactosemia
- OA, MCADD

Treatment:
- IV dextrose 2ml/kg 10%
- Followed by infusion

Mucopolysaccharidosis

- A metabolic disorder due to defects in Glycosaminoglycan's metabolism.
- Macromolecules accumulate & stored in different tissues (liver, spleen, heart, connective tissue).

- **Hunter:**
    - Iduronate sulphatase deficiency
    - X linked recessive
- **Hurler :**
    - α-L-iduronidase deficiency
    - Autosomal recessive
    - Corneal clouding
- **Sanfilipo:**
    - Severe mental retardation
- **Morquio:**
    - Skeletal deformities

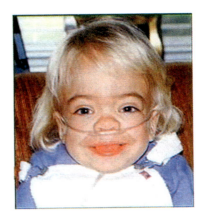

(Increased level of Glycosaminoglycan's, haptan, dermatan sulphate in urine)

Febrile Convulsions

1. It is common in children = 1:20
2. Positive Family history
3. Occurs usually at 6 months – 3 years
4. Tends to recur
5. Risk of epilepsy is 1%
6. Always associated with fever

Sudden infant death syndrome

- Unexplained death of infants before 1 year of age
- 1:2000 live births

Risk factors:

1. 1st 3 months of life
2. Prone sleep
3. Preterm
4. Inborn errors of metabolism
5. Parental smoking
6. Low maternal age
7. High birth order
8. Low birth weight
9. Over-heating, over-warping
10. Soft sleeping surfaces
11. Bed sharing with parents

Management:

1. Inform consultant immediately
2. Take the infant to the ER
3. Start resuscitation
4. Parents can attend
5. Discuss duration of resuscitation with the parents
6. Break bad news

After this

- Complete physical examination
- Investigations:
  1. CBC, electrolytes, liver functions
  2. Metabolic screening
  3. Chromosomal analysis
  4. Skin and muscle biopsy
  5. Nasopharyngeal aspirates, swabs
	- Check "at risk register"
	- Skeletal survey
	- Take pictures
	- Inform coroner
	- Inform child protection team
	- Inform social services
	- Family support

Renal tubular physiology

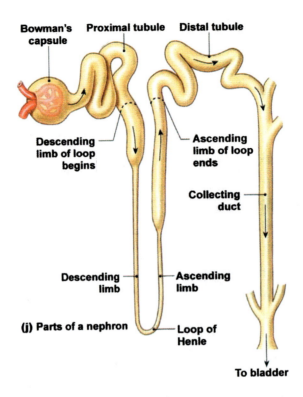

(j) Parts of a nephron

Proximal.

- ✓ 50% of Na reabsorbed (Na-K-ATPase)
- ✓ 90% of Bicarbonate reabsorbed
- ✓ 100% of Glucose reabsorbed
- ✓ 100% of Amino acids reabsorbed
- ✓ 90% of Phosphate reabsorbed
- ✓ 95% of Ca reabsorbed

Loop of Henle . 40% of Na reabsorbed (Na-K-2Cl channel)

Distal tubule   5% of Na reabsorbed

Collecting Duct   2% of Na reabsorbed in exchange with K
H+ is secreted

Electrolytes disturbance

Hyponatremia
Na < 130   Severe < 120 mmol/L

- ↑ Water in excess of Na
  - Acute renal failure
  - SIADH
  - Excess water intake (polydipsia)

Treatment: water restriction

- ↓ Na
  - Diuretics
  - ATN
  - CAH
  - Gastroenteritis
  - Cystic fibrosis

Treatment: Rehydration + Na deficits (140-Na) x 0.65 x kg

Hypernatremia
Na > 150 mmol/L

- ↓ Water
  - Diabetes insipidus
  - Diabetic ketoacidosis
  - Diarrhea, vomiting

Treatment: hydration, ORS

- ↑ Na:
  - Hypertonic, IV fluids
  - Salt poisoning

Treatment: of cause

Hypokalemia
K < 3.5 mmol/L

- Gastrointestinal losses
- Diuretics
- Diabetic ketoacidosis
- Fanconi, Bartter, Gitelmann
- Insulin treatment
- Salbutamol use in asthma

Hypocalcemia
- Vitamin D deficiency
  - Dietary, liver & renal disease
- Hypoparathyroidism
- Pseudo-Hypoparathyroidism
- Metabolic & respiratory alkalosis
- Renal failure

Hyperkalemia
K > 4.5 mmol/L

- Acute/chronic renal failure
- Metabolic acidosis
- Rhabdomyolysis/Tumor lysis syndrome
- CAH, Adrenal insufficiency
- K sparing diuretics

ECG: Peak T, prolonged PR wide QRS, VT, VF *see page 237*

Treatment
- Ca Gluconate
- Ca resonium
- Salbutamol
- Glucose/insulin

Renal tubular acidosis

	Type I distal	Type II Proximal
Mechanism	Impaired excretion of H+ Urine is never acidic ↓ K	Impaired reabsorption of bicarbonate Urine can be acidic Normal or ↓K
Causes	Primary Nephrocalcinosis Obstructive Uropathy Amphotericin, Cyclosporine	Primary Fanconi syndrome
Presentation	Nephrocalcinosis Hypokalemia	Vomiting Growth failure
NH4Cl intake	No acidic urine	Acidic urine
Treatment	NaHCO3	NaHCO3 (large doses)

Fanconi syndrome:

Causes: WCTLG (Wilson, Cystinosis, Tyrosinemia, Lowe syndrome, Galactosemia)

Proximal tubule dysfunction
- Glucose → glycosuria
- Phosphate → hypophosphatemia
- Na → Polyuria, polydipsia
- HCO3 → proximal renal tubular acidosis

Cystinosis:
- Autosomal Recessive disorder
- Defective transport of cysteine out of lysosomes
- Presented with Fanconi syndrome, renal failure, hepatomegaly, diabetes mellitus, CNS affection
- ↑ White cell cysteine level
- Treatment with cysteamine

Glomerulonephritis

Renal syndromes:

- Nephrotic syndrome
- Nephritic syndrome
- Hematuria/proteinuria
- Rapidly progressive crescentic glomerulonephritis

1. Acute post-streptococcal glomerulonephritis

- Reddish brown urine 2 weeks post streptococcal infection of skin or throat
- Renal syndromes
- Throat swab, anti-streptolysin O, biopsy
- C3, C4 ↓

2. Henoch schonlein purpura

3. IgA Nephropathy

- Micro or macroscopic hematuria
- Respiratory infection (concurrent)
- Renal syndromes

4. SLE

- Renal syndromes
- ↓ C3, C4

5. Shunt Nephritis

- ↓ C3, C4

Criteria for SLE

4 out of 11
1. Malar rash
2. Discoid rash
3. Photosensitivity
4. Oral ulcers
5. Serositis: pleuritis, pericarditis
6. Renal disorder: proteinuria
7. Neurologic disorder: seizure, psychosis
8. Hematologic disorder: neutropenia, thrombocytopenia, anemia
9. Arthritis
10. Immune : anti-DS DNA, anti-Smooth muscle antibodies
11. Anti-nuclear antibody (ANA)

Urinary tract infection

- Girls are affected more than boys but before 6 months boys are more.
- Infants are having the following specific features:
    - most vulnerable to renal damage
    - fever
    - non-specific symptoms

Presentation:

< 3 months:
- Fever, vomiting, lethargy, poor feeding, failure to thrive

< 3 months:
- Fever, dysuria, abdominal pain, loin pain, poor feeding, vomiting

Risk Factors for UTI:
- Poor urine flow
- VUR
- Evidence of spinal lesion
- Previous UTI
- Constipation
- Abdominal mass
- Recurrent fever

Investigation:

Collection of urine:
- Clean catch
- Urinary pads
- Catheters or suprapubic aspiration

Infants < 3 months	3 months-3 years	older >3 years
↓	↓	↓
Microscopy & culture	microscopy & culture	dipstick

Microscopy:

	Pyuria	Bacteria
UTI	+ve	+ve
UTI	−ve	+ve
Start Abs if clinically suggesting UTI	+ve	−ve
No UTI	−ve	−ve

Dipstick:

	Leukocyte esterase	Nitrate
UTI	+ve	+ve
UTI	−ve	+ve
Start Abs if clinically suggesting UTI	+ve	−ve
No UTI	−ve	−ve

Management:

- < 3 months   IV ABs
- \> 3 months with pyelonephritis   Oral or IV ABs for 7 days
- \> 3 months with cystitis   Oral ABs for 3 days

Prophylaxis is not routinely recommended after 1st attack

Imaging:

- <6 months   U.S, DMSA, MCUG
  - If responds to ABs within 48 hours then U.S only after 6 weeks
- 6 months – 3 years.   US, DMSA   If atypical or recurrent
- \>3 years   U.S, DMSA   If recurrent UTI

                             MCUG if: abnormality in US, DMSA, recurrent UTI + Family history

Prevention:

- Clean intermittent catheterization, plenty of fluids, Cranberry, yoghurt
- Prevent constipation

Nocturnal enuresis

Important points in History taking

1. **Pattern:**
   - How many times/night
   - How many nights/week
   - What time at night
   - Volume of urine

2. **Day time:**
   - Is he/she frequently passing urine at day (> 7 times or < 4 times?)
   - Is there urgency of micturition?
   - Any abdominal pain or strain
   - Any pain on passing urine

3. **Toilet Pattern:**
   - Does he/she avoid using certain toilets?
   - Go to toilet > or < than his peers

4. **Fluid intake**
   - How much he/she drinks per day?
   - Do parent restrict fluids?

5. **Comorbidities:**
   - UTI
   - Constipation
   - DM
   - Behavioral or emotional problems

6. **Social**
   - Do you need special sleeping arrangement?
   - Impact of bedwetting to child & parent
   - What hope do parent think treatment will achieve
   - What is their priority (short term or long term)

Management:

1. Adequate fluid intake
2. Avoid caffeine based drinks
3. Healthy diet
4. Regular toilet use during day (4-7 times)

If after the above

Some dry night	No response	Short & rapid onset is priority
		Alarm is undesirable
↓	↓	↓
Reward system	Alarm system	Desmopressin treatment

Indication for urinalysis:

1. Recent bedwetting
2. Daytime symptoms
3. Ill child
4. History suggesting UTI
5. History suggesting DM

Vesicoureteral Reflux

Presentation:

2 Groups
- Hydronephrosis
- Urinary tract infection

- Non-specific symptoms
- Abdominal pain
- Voiding symptoms
- Incomplete emptying
- Double micturition

Grades:

- Grade I — Reflux into ureter with no dilatation
- Grade II — Reflux into pelvis & calyces
- Grade III — Reflux with mild dilatation
- Grade IV — Reflux with moderate dilatation
- Grade V — Reflux with severe dilatation

Grade 4, 5 will need surgical intervention mostly.

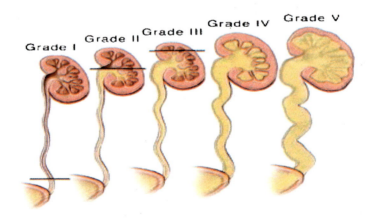

Chronic renal failure

Causes:

1. Renal Scarring: multiple UTI, VUR
2. Hereditary: Polycystic kidney, Alport syndrome, Cystinosis
3. Congenital dysplasia
4. Henoch schonlein purpura
5. SLE
6. Tumors

Investigations:

1. CBC
2. Electrolytes, Creatinine, Urea, Bicarbonate
3. Ca, PO4, Alkaline Phosphatase
4. Protein, Albumin
5. Wrist X-ray
6. Renal US
7. Monitor BP, urine analysis

Complications:

Issue	Treatment
Hypertension	B-blocker, furosemide
Metabolic acidosis	
Growth failure	Growth Hormone
Anemia	Erythropoietin
Renal Osteodystrophy	Vitamin D, PO4 restriction
Uremia (nausea, anorexia)	Protein restriction
Seizures	Anti-epileptics

Renal transplant

1. Transplant is the main aim before dialysis.

2. Living donor is better

    - Better long term survival
    - Transplant with no dialysis

3. Should be HLA (A, B, DR) matched

4. Immunosuppressive drugs

    - Prednisone
    - Tacrolimus
    - Azathioprine

5. Children must be > 10 kg

6. Children must be immune to TB, chicken pox, measles

7. Complication.

    - Surgical complication
    - Rejection
    - Infection
    - Drug toxicity
    - Lymphoproliferative disorders

Renal Osteodystrophy

- Failure to convert Vitamin D to active Vitamin D
- Decreased Ca absorption
- Decreased Ca level
- Increased PTH
- Bone demineralization, Ca resorption
- Increased PO4 level, Decreased PO4 excretion

Treatment:

- Vitamin D
- PO4 restriction on diet
- PO4 binders (Ca carbonate)

Chronic Diarrhea

Causes:

- Infection (giardia)
- Secondary lactose intolerance post infection
- Cow milk protein allergy
- Cystic fibrosis
- Coeliac disease
- Immunodeficiency

Warning signs:

- Failure to thrive
- Bloody diarrhea
- Systemic upset
- Frequent and massive

Headache

Types of Headache:

1. **Primary**
   - Migraine
   - Tension
   - Cluster
2. **Secondary**
   - Trauma to head or neck
   - Vascular or non-vascular
   - Infection or psychogenic
3. **Cranial neuralgia, facial pain**

Investigation:

- CBC, PT, PTT
- Lumbar puncture
- CT, MRI Brain

Special tests:

Fundoscopy – visual fields – blood pressure – head circumference

Headache warning sign:

1. Awakening from sleep
2. Morning headache
3. Occipital pain
4. Increasing severity
5. Increases with cough, straining
6. Change in behavior and school performance

Management: *see page 54*

- Most important: life style changes, (sleep   exercise – tension   stress – diet)
- Monitoring of school performance
- Simple analgesics and prophylaxis in case of migraine

Tics

Characteristics:

- Involuntary, abnormal movements which are done unintentionally and can be suppressed over a period of time but return back.

- Common between school children & can grow out of it with time.

- Examples. blinking, coughing, lip biting.

➢ Increased with physical stress, exhaustion, heat, emotional stress.

➢ No investigation and diagnosed clinically

Advices

1. Don't draw attention.

2. Seek advice if
    - Increased severity
    - Associated with aggression
    - Depression
    - Interfere with daily activity

3. Relaxation techniques may help.

Neurofibromatosis Type I

- One of the neurocutaneous syndromes = CNS manifestation + Skin diseases
- AD inheritance and 50% are DE novo
- The protein affected is the Neurofibromin, Gene is located on chromosome 17

Diagnosis: 2 or more of

1) 1st degree relative
2) Optic glioma
3) Axillary freckling
4) Osseous lesions
5) 2 or more Lisch nodules
6) 2 or more neurofibroma
7) 6 or more café-au-Lait spots

Complication:

- Learning difficulties
- Macrocephaly
- Short stature

Renal artery stenosis
Scoliosis
Spinal cord compression

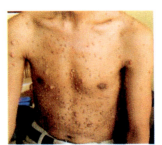

Neurofibroma

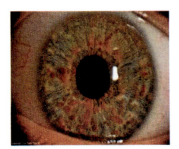

Lisch nodules

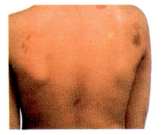

Café Au Lait patches

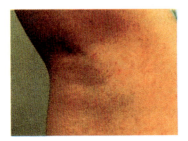

Axillary frecklings

Ataxia

Ataxia may be due to sensory or cerebellar lesion

Causes:

Acute	Intermittent	Chronic

- Infectious:
   o Chicken pox
   o Measles
- Tumors
- Metabolic disorders
- Drugs:
   o Phenytoin
	- Migraine
	- Epilepsy
		- Friedreich's ataxia
		- Ataxia telangiectasia
		- Wilson's disease
		- Vitamin E deficiency
		- Encephalopathy

Friedreich's Ataxia

- Autosomal recessive disorder, due to pyramidal tract dysfunction
- Signs of cerebellar degeneration and peripheral neuropathy

Signs:

- **Ataxia / Romberg's positive / extensor planters / loss of position & vibration sense**
- Nystagmus
- Pes cavus
- Kyphoscoliosis
- Hypertrophic cardiomyopathy

Ataxia Telangiectasia

- Autosomal recessive disorder
- Cerebellar ataxia associated with conjunctival and ear telangiectasia
- Prone to develop malignancy
- Lab works shows high levels of Alpha-fetoprotein and low levels of IgA & IgG

Tuberous sclerosis

- Autosomal dominant disorder due to mutations at chromosomes 9 & 16
- 70% are new mutations

Presentation:

Skin	Eye	CNS	Kidney	Cardiac
Adenoma sebaceum Asche leaf macules Shagreen patches Café-au-lait spots Periungual fibromas	Hamartomas Retinal phakomas	Astrocytoma Glioma Hydrocephalus	Renal angiomas	Rhabdomyoma

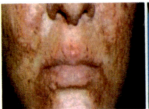 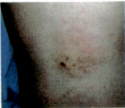 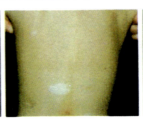 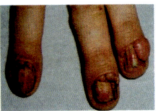

Adenoma sebaceum   **Shagreen patches**   **Asche leaf macules**   **Periungual fibromas**

Complications:

- Seizures, infantile spasms (Hypsarrythmia) *see page 148*
- Learning difficulties
- Autism

Investigations:

- Woods lamp to detect skin lesions
- Monitor blood pressure
- ECG & echocardiography
- EEG
- CT or MRI

Management: *see page 54*

- Multidisciplinary team approach
- Referral to all concerned specialties

Wilson's disease

- This is a disease due to abnormal Copper metabolism
- It results from accumulation of Copper due to decreased binding Ceruloplasmin
- It is an autosomal recessive disorder with mutations in chromosome 13

Presentation:

Hepatic

- Jaundice
- Elevated liver enzymes
- Acute & chronic liver failure
- Acute hepatitis
- Cirrhosis & Pulmonary hypertension

CNS

- School deterioration
- Mood changes
- Tremors
- Dysarthria & Incoordination

Others

- Cataract
- Hemolytic anemia
- Cardiac problems

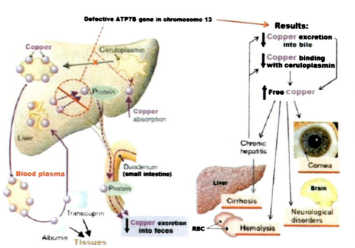

Diagnosis:

- Decreased ceruloplasmin
- Elevated urinary Copper
- Elevated Liver Copper
- Kayser – Fleisher ring

Treatment:

Penicillamine - Liver transplantation

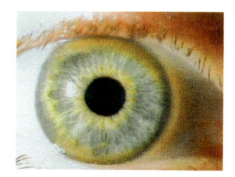

Epilepsy

Abnormal excessive electric discharge from cerebral neurons.

Classification of seizures:

| Partial || Generalized |
simple	complex	
	Loss of consciousness	Absence Tonic Clonic Tonic clonic Atonic Myoclonic

Classification of epileptic syndromes:

Localized	Generalized	Unclassified
Benign Rolandic (nocturnal, male>female, affects upper limb) Temporal Parietal Frontal Occipital	Benign familial Benign neonatal Juvenile myoclonic (on wakening from sleep) Infantile spasm	Neonatal Landau - kleffner

Investigation:
- EEG, Sleep EEG, sleep deprived EEG
- MRI if treatment failed

Important points in history:

Before attack	During attack	After attack
Witness Visual, olfactory, auditory hallucination Pallor, sweating, nausea, vomiting Triggers: noise, stress, light	Description Duration, how terminated Site Urine, stool incontinence	Degree of alertness & consciousness

Management of Epilepsy

See page 54

Main points:

1. Side effect
2. Start with one drug
3. Keep 2 years maintenance (epileptic free)
4. Withdraw gradually
5. Drug level monitoring
6. Interaction with other medications

Type of seizure	Medication	Main side effects
Partial Generalized	Carbamazepine	Ataxia, neutropenia, thrombocytopenia, rash
All Seizures	Na valproate	Nausea, vomiting, abdominal pain, hair loss, liver toxicity
Partial Infantile spasm	Vigabatrin	Visual filed disorder
Absence	Ethosaximide	GIT disorder
All Seizures	Phenytoin	Nausea, vomiting, peripheral neuropathy, rash

Status epilepticus:

IV access

Step1 : Lorazepam or diazepam
Step 2: Rectal paraldehyde
Step 3: phenytoin

No IV access:

Step1   Rectal diazepam
Step 2. Intraosseous diazepam

Last step: Anesthesia

Head injury

Mild closed head Injury	Severe closed head Injury	Non-accidental (shaken baby syndrome)
Crying Vomiting Lethargy	Major loss of consciousness	Impaired consciousness History inconsistent with injury Shock Bruises Fractures Retinal hemorrhage

Clinical Assessment:

1. Level of consciousness
2. Respiratory Pattern
3. Pupil size, reaction
4. CSF leakage
5. Focal signs
6. Assessment of cervical spine

Management:

- Airway, breathing, circulation support
- X-ray spine
- CT Brain
- Assess intracranial pressure

Complication:

- Headache
- Epilepsy
- Learning disabilities
- Motor deficits

Glasgow coma scale

Eye opening

- Spontaneous   4
- Speech   3
- Pain   2
- None   1

Verbal Response

- Oriented   5
- Words   4
- Inappropriate words   3
- Cries   2
- None   1

Motor response

- Obeys commands   6
- Localizes pain   5
- Withdraws to pain   4
- Flexion to pain   3
- Extension to pain   2
- None   1

Total: 15

Severe: ≤ 8

Moderate: 9-12

EEG patterns

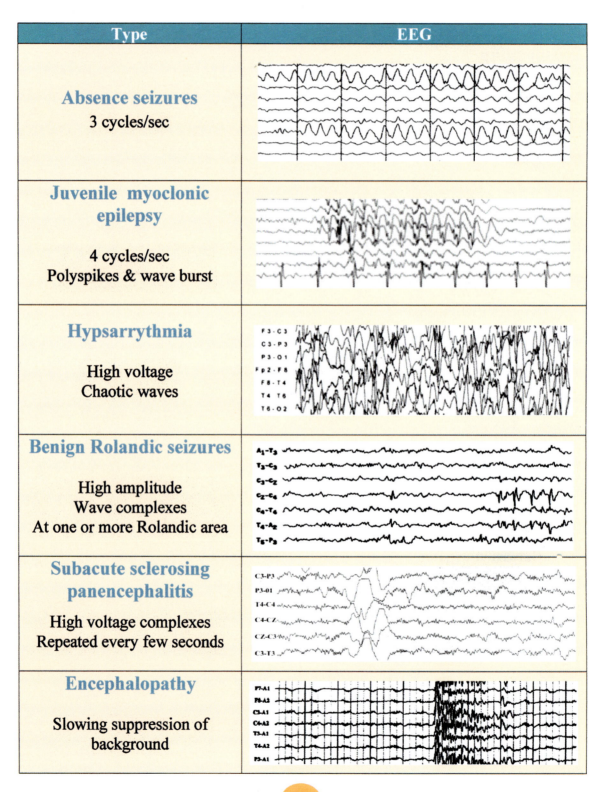

Type	EEG
Absence seizures 3 cycles/sec	
Juvenile myoclonic epilepsy 4 cycles/sec Polyspikes & wave burst	
Hypsarrythmia High voltage Chaotic waves	
Benign Rolandic seizures High amplitude Wave complexes At one or more Rolandic area	
Subacute sclerosing panencephalitis High voltage complexes Repeated every few seconds	
Encephalopathy Slowing suppression of background	

Hypersensitivity reactions

	Type I	Type II	Type III	Type IV
Mediator	IgE	IgG, IgM	IgG	T cell
Mechanism	Mast cell degranulation	Complement activation	Immune complex	T helper 1,2 Cytotoxic T cell
Conditions	Asthma Food allergy Anaphylaxis	Hemolytic arthus reaction	Serum sickness Erythema nodosum	Tuberculin test Chronic asthma Contact dermatitis

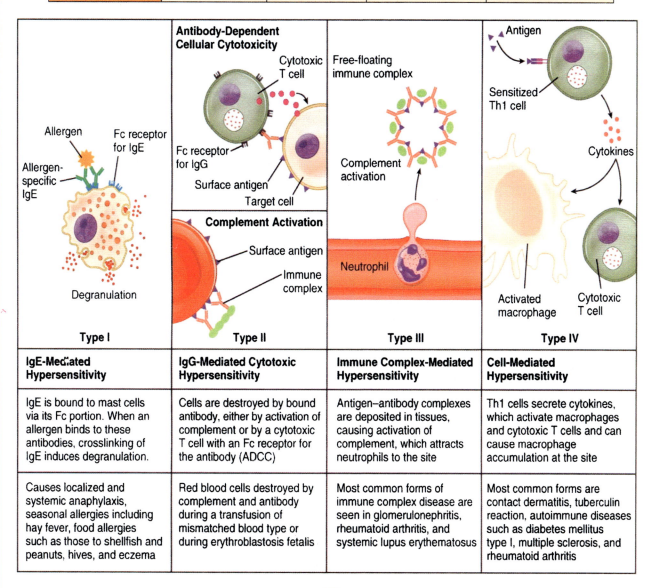

Type I	Type II	Type III	Type IV
IgE-Mediated Hypersensitivity	**IgG-Mediated Cytotoxic Hypersensitivity**	**Immune Complex-Mediated Hypersensitivity**	**Cell-Mediated Hypersensitivity**
IgE is bound to mast cells via its Fc portion. When an allergen binds to these antibodies, crosslinking of IgE induces degranulation.	Cells are destroyed by bound antibody, either by activation of complement or by a cytotoxic T cell with an Fc receptor for the antibody (ADCC)	Antigen–antibody complexes are deposited in tissues, causing activation of complement, which attracts neutrophils to the site	Th1 cells secrete cytokines, which activate macrophages and cytotoxic T cells and can cause macrophage accumulation at the site
Causes localized and systemic anaphylaxis, seasonal allergies including hay fever, food allergies such as those to shellfish and peanuts, hives, and eczema	Red blood cells destroyed by complement and antibody during a transfusion of mismatched blood type or during erythroblastosis fetalis	Most common forms of immune complex disease are seen in glomerulonephritis, rheumatoid arthritis, and systemic lupus erythematosus	Most common forms are contact dermatitis, tuberculin reaction, autoimmune diseases such as diabetes mellitus type I, multiple sclerosis, and rheumatoid arthritis

Anaphylaxis

- **Anaphylaxis:** occurs due to release of histamine causing local reaction or wide spread manifestations
- **Anaphylactic shock:** this is simply a circulatory collapse

Spectrum of manifestations:

- Fever
- Rash & Urtecaria
- Tachycardia & Tachypnea
- Laryngeal edema & Stridor
- Hypotension
- Respiratory depression
- Renal failure
- Death

Management: if in shock then start boluses of normal saline and IV adrenaline infusion

- Remove the antigen
- Airway, respiratory and cardiac support
- Oxygen therapy
- Adrenaline

Then if

Complete obstruction
Air way insertion

Partial obstruction
Nebulized adrenaline
Nebulized salbutamol
IV hydrocortisone

EPIPEN: Calm   Remove Cap   Right angle at thigh   Press   Wait 10 sec - Massage for 5 sec

Transfusion reactions

Spectrum:

- **Hemolytic Reaction (ABO incompatibility)**
    - Antibodies from recipient react with donor antigen
    - Hemolysis, DIC, Renal failure

- **Bacterial Infection**

- **Non-hemolytic febrile reaction**
    - Fever, chills, rigors
    - From cytokine production by donor leukocytes

- **Anaphylactic Reaction**
    - Hypotension, bronchospasm, rash, urticaria, laryngeal edema

- **Transfusion related acute lung injury (TRALI)**
    - Donor antibodies react with recipient leukocyte
    - Cough, breathlessness
    - CXR. bilateral lung infiltrates

Poisoning

Paracetamol	Iron	TCA	Aspirin	Lead
Clinical picture				

1 – Nausea, vomiting, abdominal pain
2 – Hepatic necrosis
3 – Liver failure
	I – Nausea, vomiting, abdominal pain, hematemesis
	II Apparent recovery
	III – Hypoglycemia
	IV – Liver failure
		- Unconsciousness
		- Convulsion
		- Arrhythmia
		- Hypotension
		- Respiratory depression
		  Pupil dilatation
		- Urine retention
		- Dry mouth
			I – Respiratory Alkalosis
			II – Hypokalemia
			III – Hypokalemia
			  Dehydration
			  Lactic Acidosis
			  Pulmonary edema
			  Respiratory depression
				- Failure to thrive
				- Anemia (Microcytic-hypochromic)
				- CNS: confusion, dizziness, coma, altered behavior
				- Abdomen: nausea, vomiting, constipation

Management				
Resuscitate		**Poison Unit**		**Level**
-Activated Charcoal 4 hours -Acetyl cysteine 24 hours -Level at 4 hours	X-ray abdomen No Desferal oral In stomach Desferal + lavage In intestine Desferal + laxative >60mg/kg IV Deferoxamine	- NaHCO₃ - Hydration - Alkalization	- Activated Charcoal - Gastric lavage - Hydration - Alkalization	Mild: d-penicillamine Moderate: EDTA Severe: EDTA+ dimercaprol

Hirschsprung disease

- It is absence if ganglion cells in the myenteric plexus of the distal bowel
- It is associated with Down syndrome and other congenital anomalies
- Usually presented in infancy but can occur in childhood and present as functional constipation

Diagnosis:

- Rectal biopsy
- Histochemistry: excessive acetylcholinesterase activity

Management:

- Surgical excision
- Temporary colostomy, Pull through

Hepatomegaly & Splenomegaly

Causes:

Hepatomegaly	Splenomegaly
▪ **Infection:** o Hepatitis A o Hepatitis B o Epstein – Barr virus ▪ **Malignancy:** o Liver tumors o Leukemia, lymphoma, neuroblastoma ▪ **Storage disease:** o Cystic fibrosis o Gaucher's disease o Glycogen storage disease o Niemann – pick syndrome ▪ **Others:** o Congestive heart failure o Wilson's disease o Alpha 1 antitrypsin deficiency	▪ **Infection:** o Epstein – Barr virus o Septicemia o Malaria ▪ **Malignancy** o Leukemia, lymphoma o Metastatic tumors ▪ **Storage disease:** o Gaucher's disease ▪ **Others** o Systemic lupus erythematosus o Juvenile idiopathic arthritis o Portal hypertension o Cirrhosis ▪ **Hematology** o Sickle cell anemia o Thalassemia o Spherocytosis

Glycogen storage disease

Type I – Von Gierke's disease

Autosomal recessive disorder

Due to reduced activity of glucose-6-phosphatase enzyme

Diagnosis:

- Liver biopsy
- Enzymatic activity
- Genotyping

Presentation:

1. Asymptomatic hepatomegaly
2. Hypoglycemia
3. Lactic acidosis
4. Short stature
5. Doll-like facies
6. Nephromegaly
7. Renal calculi
8. Hepatoma
9. Platelets dysfunction
10. Intellectual impairment

Type II (Pompe disease):

- Muscle affection

Type III

- Muscle affection   /   Hepatomegaly

Type IV

   Hepatomegaly

Type V

- Muscle affection

Portal hypertension

Causes:

POST
- Budd – Chiari syndrome
- Right ventricular failure
- Constrictive pericarditis

HEPATIC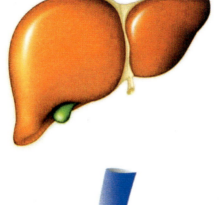
- **Pre-sinusoidal:** tumor, cyst
- **Sinusoidal:** fibrosis, cirrhosis
- **Post-sinusoidal:** veno-occlusive disease

PRE
- Portal vein thrombosis

Presentation:
- Failure to thrive
- Splenomegaly
- Caput medusa
- Ascites

Complications:
- GI hemorrhage (varices, hemorrhoids, and encephalopathy)
- Hypersplenism (anemia, thrombocytopenia, leukopenia)

Bilirubin metabolism

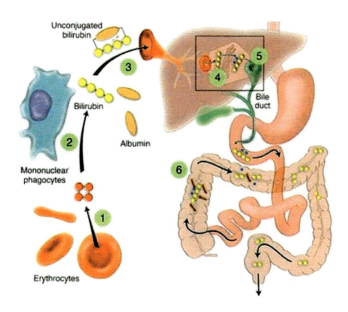

1. Hemoglobin gives rise to **heme** and **globin**
2. Heme is catabolized to **unconjugated bilirubin** in the RES
3. Unconjugated bilirubin binds to **albumin**
4. Uptake of unconjugated bilirubin by hepatocytes then unconjugated bilirubin is converted to **Conjugated bilirubin** by **glucuronosyl transferase enzyme**
5. Conjugated bilirubin is secreted in bile & enters duodenum
6. In the bowel

       Conjugated Bilirubin
    ⬇   ⬇

Unconjugated   Glucuronic acid
⬇

Excreted in stool

Some reabsorbed back to liver (enterohepatic circulation)

Unconjugated hyperbilirubinemia

Same causes as neonatal jaundice

- **Increased production (hemolysis)**
    - RH incompatibility
    - ABO Incompatibility
    - Spherocytosis
    - Elliptocytosis
    - G6PD deficiency
    - Pyruvate Kinase deficiency
    - SCA
    - Thalassemia

- **Decreased uptake by hepatocytes**
    - Breast Milk Jaundice

- **Decreased conjugation**
    - Physiological jaundice
    - Crigler Najjar
        - I-severe
        - II- moderate decrease of glucuronosyl transferase enzyme
    - Gilbert disease: mild decrease of glucuronosyl transferase enzyme

- **Others:**
    - Infection
    - Drug induced
    - Cystic fibrosis
    - Pyloric Stenosis

Conjugated hyperbilirubinemia

- **Infection:**
    - Bacteria
        - UTI
        - Syphilis
        - TB
        - Septicemia
    - Viral
        - CMV
        - Herpes
        - EBV
        - HIV
        - Hepatitis A, B
- **Metabolic:**
    - Galactosemia
    - GSD
    - Tyrosinemia
    - Niemann pick syndrome
    - Zellweger's Syndrome
- **Endocrine:**
    - Hyperthyroidism
- **Others:**
    - Down syndrome
    - Cystic fibrosis
    - Wilson's disease
    - Dubin Johnson
    - Rotor syndrome

Most Common
- Neonatal hepatitis
- Intrahepatic Biliary atresia (Allagille syndrome)
- Extrahepatic Biliary atresia
- Alpha 1 antitrypsin deficiency

Biliary atresia

- 1 16000 live birth
- Female are more affected than males

Types:

 I. Obliteration of common bile duct
 II. Obliteration of hepatic duct
 III. Obliteration of whole extrahepatic biliary tree

Diagnosis:

- Hepatobiliary US
- Radionuclide imaging
- Liver biopsy
- Exploration & cholangiography

Treatment:

- Kasai operation within 60 days of birth
- Fat soluble vitamins
- Complication. Ascending cholangitis 50%

Prognosis:

80% require transplantation at 20 years of age

Cirrhosis

Chronic liver disease signs:

1. Palmar erythema
2. Spider nevi
3. Gynecomastia
4. Pallor
5. Clubbing
6. Female hair distribution

Complication of Cirrhosis:

1. Portal hypertension
2. Hepato-renal disease – renal failure
3. Hepato-pulmonary disease – Pulmonary hypertension
4. Hepatic encephalopathy
5. Hepatoma
6. Bleeding, Coagulopathy
7. Infection, Peritonitis
8. Malnutrition, Growth failure

Management:

- Identify & treat cause
- Identify & treat complication
- Diet:
    - ↑ protein, vitamins, minerals
    - ↓ salt ± diuretics
- Bleeding:
    - Fresh frozen Plasma, Blood transfusion
- Peritonitis:
    - Antibiotics
- Encephalopathy:
    - Neomycin
    - Lactulose
- Liver transplant

Management of liver failure

1. **Refer to liver Center**

2. **Ventilation:**
   - Respiratory failure
   - Encephalopathy

3. **Monitoring**
   - O2 saturation
   - Neuro observation
   - Vital signs
   - Acid base balance
   - CBC
   - Fluid balance

4. **Blood Products**
   - Fresh frozen plasma if bleeding
   - Keep Platelets > 50,000

5. **Drugs:**
   - H2 blocker, proton pump inhibitor
   - Lactulose
   - Neomycin

6. **Nutrition**
   - Enteral or parental

7. **Specific:**
   - Paracetamol toxicity →acetylcysteine
   - Iron toxicity → chelation

8. **Liver Transplant**

Liver transplant

Indication:

- Acute Liver Failure
- Chronic Liver Failure
- Tumors
- Metabolic Disease

Contraindication:

- Severe sepsis
- Metastatic tumors
- Irreversible extrahepatic damage (brain, CVS)

Source:

Decreased donor   or   Living related donor

Type:

Whole liver   or   Segmental graft

Immunosuppression by:

- Steroids
- Cyclosporine
- Tacrolimus
- mTOR inhibitor
- Azathioprine

Complication:

Early	1st week	Late
Graft failure	Rejection	Immune suppression
Drug side effect	Sepsis	EBV, Hepatitis A
	Biliary leak	Portal vein thrombosis

Hormone physiology of anterior pituitary gland

Gonadotrophins:

LH	Stimulate testosterone production (male)
	Stimulate steroidogenesis (female)
FSH	↑ Mass of seminiferous tubules (male)
	Convert testosterone → estrogen (female)

GnRH: ↑ LH, FSH
Inhibin: ↓ FSH

Growth Hormone:

- Direct Effect on carbohydrate and lipid metabolism
- Effect mediated by IGF-1 which.
  - ↑ Protein synthesis
  - ↑ DNA, RNA, lipogenesis

GHRH: ↑ GH

Somatostatin: ↓ GH

Prolactin:

- Induction of lactation, ↓ menses

Dopamine: ↓ Prolactin

TSH:

- Increase production of thyroid hormone

ACTH:

- Stimulate adrenal cortex to produce cortisone

CRH: ↑ ACTH release

Diabetes Insipidus (DI)

- Insufficient ADH which will cause polyuria, polydipsia
- If decreased water intake → hypernatremic dehydration

Causes:

Central
- Craniopharyngioma
- LCH
- Germinoma
- Tumor

Renal
- X-linked nephrogenic DI

Diagnosis Water deprivation test

1. Weight child
2. Deprive water intake for 7 hours
3. Stop the test if
   - Weight decreased by 5%
   - Dehydration
   - Osmolality > 295 osm/L
4. Diagnosis of DI if plasma osmolality > 290 osm/L

5. Give **DDAVP**
   - This will normally increase Urine concentration
   - Inability to concentrate urine will confirm Nephrogenic DI

Treatment

- DDAVP (desmopressin) spray or tablet

(SIADH):

- Water retention, hyponatremia
- Caused by Pneumonia meningitis, trauma, malignancy, VCR, CTX
- Treatment cause, fluid balance, fluid restriction

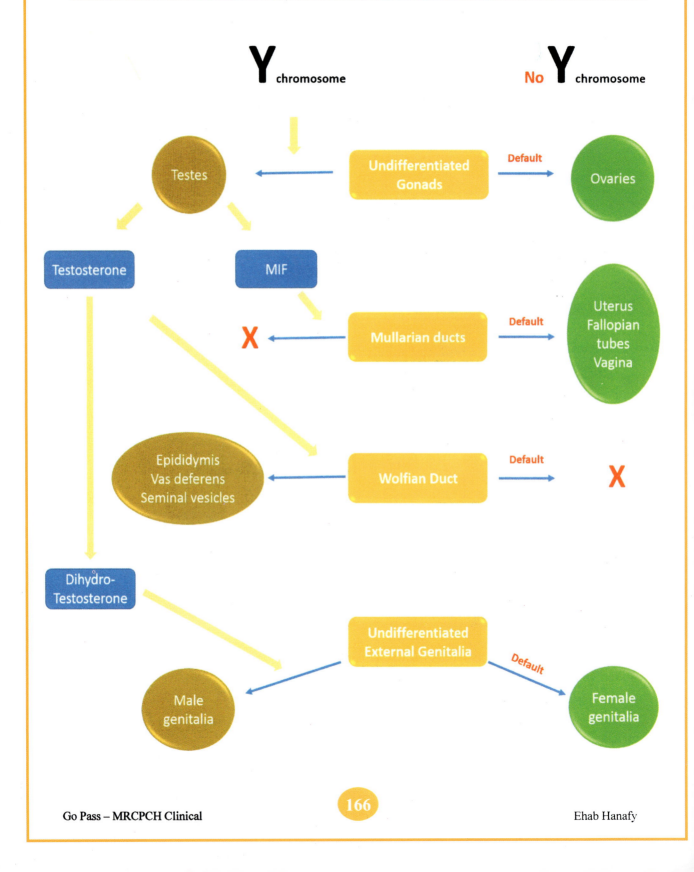

Precocious puberty

- < 9 years in boys and < 8 years in girls
- In girls there is usually no cause
- In male it is almost always pathological

Types:

Gonadotropin dependent	Gonadotropin independent
Idiopathic	McCune Albright
CNS tumors	Testicular/Ovarian tumors
Septo-optic dysplasia	Liver or adrenal tumors
Neurofibromatosis	

Investigations:

- Estradiol, testosterone
- 17 hydroxyprogesterone
- LHRH stimulation test
- MRI Brain
- CT abdomen
- Pelvic US
- Bone Age

Management:

Gonadotrophin-releasing hormone agonists (GnRHa)

Delayed puberty

- In boys it is usually constitutional
- In girls it is mostly pathologic

Causes:

1. Constitutional
2. Pituitary Disorder
3. Anorexia Nervosa
4. Kallman Syndrome
5. Hypothyroidism
6. Gonadal dysgenesis

Investigations:

- Estrogen, testosterone
- LHRH test
- LH, FSH
- Pelvic US
- Karyotyping

Management:

- Constitutional. reassurance/androgen
- Others.
    - Treatment of Cause
    - Induction of Puberty

Ambiguous Genitalia

Virialized Female	Inadequately virilized male	True Hermaphrodite
CAH	Gonadal dysgenesis	
Ovarian, adrenal tumor	LH Deficiency	
Androgen of fetal origin	Leydig cell hypoplasia	
Androgen of maternal origin	5-alpha reductase deficiency	

Investigation:

- LH, FSH
- Testosterone
- 17 OH progesterone
- Karyotyping
- Pelvic US

Management:

Multidisciplinary Approach.

- Endocrine
- Urology
- Gynecology
- Psychology

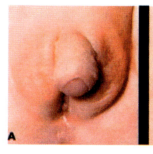 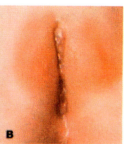

Before surgery   **After surgery**

Adrenal gland cortex

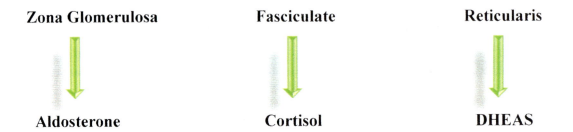

Cortisol:

- Vital role in body's stress response
- Insulin counter regulatory hormone
- Important for action of adrenaline/noradrenaline
- Important for CVS, CNS, inflammatory response

Under Control of ACTH

Mineralocorticoids (aldosterone):

- Increased Na re-absorption in exchange with K, H under control of Renin-angiotensin system

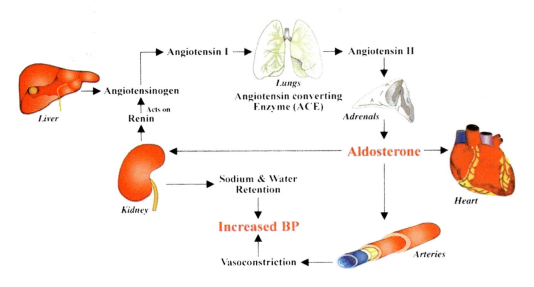

Congenital Adrenal Hyperplasia

- Most common one is 21, hydroxylase deficiency
- Leads to decreased production of cortisol, aldosterone
- Increased metabolites → androgens

Presentation:

Wide variety of presentation

1. Salt losing crisis in males
2. Virilization, ambiguous genitalia in females
3. Premature adrenarche, precocious puberty

Investigation:

- 17 OH progesterone
- ACTH, Cortisol levels
- Ultrasound Pelvis and ovaries
- Genetic testing

Treatment:

- Glucocorticoids, mineralocorticoid
- Salt replacement
- Monitor:
    - growth, BP
    - 17 OH Progesterone, salt, renin

Surgery if ambiguous genitalia

Adrenal insufficiency

Primary	Secondary
Idiopathic	ACTH deficiency
CAH	Pituitary hypoplasia
Addison disease	Tumors
Adrenal Hemorrhage	

Addison Disease:

- Autoimmune
- TB
- Adrenal leukodystrophy

Clinical picture:

- Fatigue, abdominal pain
- Collapse (salt losing crisis)

Investigation:

- Synacthen test
- 24 hours blood cortisol profile

Treatment:

- Glucocorticoids
- Mineralocorticoids

Hypoglycemia

Causes:

Decreased Production	Increased Consumption	Persistent
Counter regulatory hormone Galactosemia	Infant of diabetic mother Beckwith Weidman	Insulinoma Exogenous insulin

Investigation:

- Glucose
- Insulin
- GH
- Cortisol
- Lactate
- Free fatty acids

```
Hypoglycemia
   ↓
Ketones in urine
   ↓ No                    ↓ Yes
  FFA              ↓ Counter Regulatory hormone
 ↓    ↓            Enzyme defect in glycogenolysis
No   Yes           or gluconeogenesis
Hyperinsulinism   Fatty acid oxidation defect
```

Bone and Calcium metabolism

Ca is regulated by Vitamin D, PTH, and Calcitonin

Vitamin D

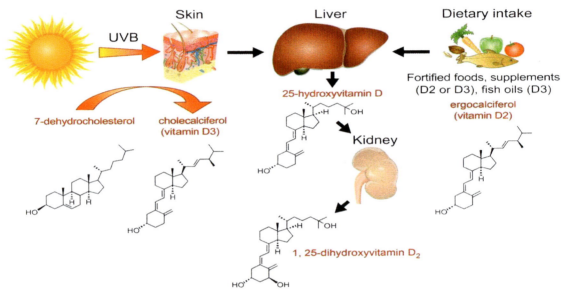

- Increases absorption of Ca
- Increases bone resorption
- Inhibits PTH secretion

PTH
- ↓ renal Ca excretion
- ↑ Ca reabsorption
- ↑ Phosphatemia
- Mobilize Ca from bones

Calcitonin
- Inhibit bone resorption

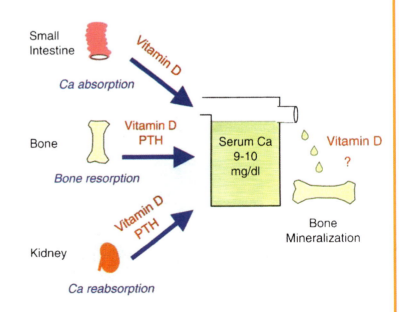

Pathophysiology of Insulin Dependent Diabetes Mellitus

- Glucose homeostasis depends mainly on insulin and glucagon
- Diabetes is a chronic metabolic disorder and in children its mainly type I IDDM
- Occurs in 20:100000 children
- Risk factors.
    - Genetic factors
    - Family history
    - Viral infection
    - As a part of syndrome (Down syndrome)
    - As a part of disease (cystic fibrosis)
- Mostly autoimmune, due to presence of antibodies against Beta cells of islets of Langerhans in pancreas

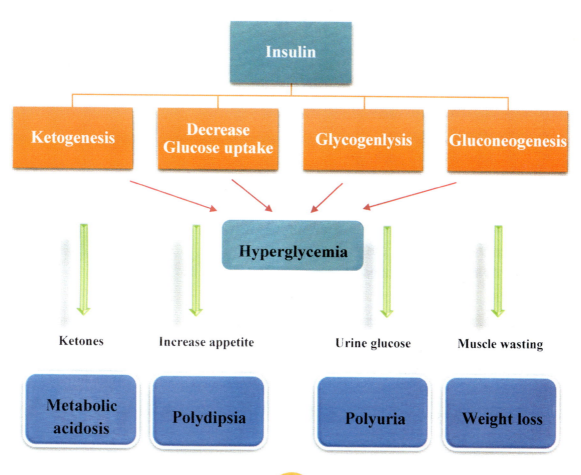

Management of Diabetes mellitus

1. **Diagnosis:**
   - Symptomatic: FBS > 7 mmol/L
   - Non-symptomatic: 2 FBS > 7, 2 times RBS > 11.1
2. **Screening:**
   1. All diabetic should be screened for depression
   2. At age of 12: screen for retinopathy
   3. Thyroid disease
   4. Coeliac disease
   5. Foot Disease
   6. Patient with cystic fibrosis should be screened annually for DM from 10 years old
3. **Lifestyle management**
4. **Continuing Management**
5. **Prevent long-term constipation**

Lifestyle Management

Delivery of Interventions:
- Educational programs
- Computer assisted packages

Depression:
- Screening & appropriate treatment
- Selective serotonin re-uptake inhibitors (SSRIs)
- Cognitive behavioral therapy
- Psychotherapy programs

Exercise:
- Maintain moderate level of physical activity

Diet:
- Reduction of weight

Smoking:
- Cessation of Smoking
- Nicotine replacement therapy

Insulin regimens

Regimens	Types of Insulin	Advantages	Disadvantages
Basal Bolus	Intermediate acting Rapid or short acting at meal time	More physiological Control what to eat & when to eat	More injections School injections
Twice a day	Mixed short, Intermediate acting	Less injection	Adjust snakes Specific meal timing
Insulin pump		Most precise control	Frequent tests Connect 24 hours Expensive set-up Risk of infection

Types of Insulin:

	Onset	Duration
Rapid acting	10-30 minutes	5 hours
Short acting	30 minutes – 1 hour	12 hours
Intermediate acting	4 hours	24 hours
Long acting	4 hours	24 hours

Obesity

- BMI > 98 Centile for age & sex
- Childhood obesity is major predictor for adulthood obesity
- Main Cause: ↑ intake and ↓ expenditure
- Needs comorbid assessment:
    - ✓ Thyroid Profile
    - ✓ Fasting blood sugar
    - ✓ Insulin Level
    - ✓ Lipid profile

Complications:

Diabetes Mellitus, Hypertension, Ischemic heart disease, Stroke, Cancer Depression, Obstructive sleep apnea, Bullying.

Causes:

Chromosomal	Endocrine	Oncologic
Prader-willi syndrome	Hypothyroidism	Pituitary tumors
Down	Cushing syndrome	
Laurence Moon Biedl	GH deficiency	
Klinefelter syndrome	Polycystic ovaries	

Management: *see page 54*

- Prevention and reduction of weight
- Exercise program
- Healthy food
- Health education

Anorexia Nervosa

- Eating disorder affecting 1% of adolescent females.
- Peak age 15-25 years

Risk Factors:

- Family history of
    - Eating disorders
    - Depression
    - Alcoholism
- Monozygotic twins 50%
- Dizygotic twins 10%
- Rigid, overprotective families
- High social class
- Low self-esteem
- Previous history of obesity

Clinical picture:

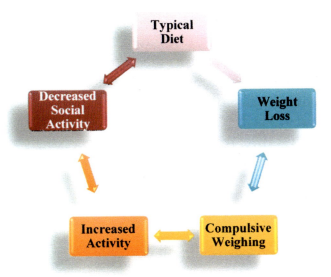

Criteria:

1. Weight loss > 15%
2. Fear of weight gain
3. Abnormal perception of body image
4. Amenorrhea

Complications:

CVS	Bradycardia, ↓BP, arrhythmia
Chest	Aspiration pneumonia
GIT	Constipation, delayed gastric emptying
Skin	Dry, thickened, lanugo hair
CNS	Cortical atrophy
Blood	↓ Platelet, anemia
Renal	↓ K, ↓ mg, metabolic alkalosis

Management: *see page 54*

- Family education
- Lifestyle changes
- Continuous monitoring of diet, exercise, weight gain
- Contact support groups & organizations
- Referral. Psychologist

  - **Specific**: Antipsychotics, antidepressants
  - Treatment of complications

Admission if weight gain at home is inappropriate.

Prognosis:

- 50% recover
- 25% recover with eating disorder
- 25% progress or die

Hyperthyroidism

- Autoimmune disease due to the production of thyroid stimulating antibodies
- Common in females
- Family history is common
- Associated with HLA DR3/B8

Symptoms:

1. Anxiety
2. Sweating
3. Heat intolerance
4. Palpitation
5. Weight loss
6. Emotional disturbance

Signs:

1. Tall stature
2. Warm hands
3. Tremors
4. Tachycardia
5. Wide pulse pressure
6. Eye signs, *see thyroid examination page 34*
7. Goiter
8. Proximal myopathy

Investigations:

- Thyroid function test; T3, T4, TSH
- Thyroid stimulating antibodies
- Bone age

Treatment:

- Medical. propranolol, carbimazole
- Radioactive iodine
- Surgical. subtotal thyroidectomy

Hypothyroidism

Causes:

Congenital	Acquired	
	Goiter	No goiter
▪ Thyroid dysgenesis ▪ Dyshormonogenesis ▪ TSH/TRH deficiency	▪ Autoimmune thyroiditis ▪ Dyshormonogenesis ▪ Iodine deficiency ▪ Malignancy	▪ Hypoplastic ▪ Post-surgical ▪ Post irradiation

Clinical picture

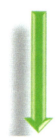
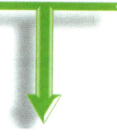

- Poor feeding
- Wide fontanelles
- Macroglossia
- Jaundice
- Constipation
- Umbilical hernia
- Developmental delay

- Poor feeding
- Increased tendency to sleep
- Cold intolerance
- Delayed teething
- Constipation
- Poor school performance

Investigations:

- Thyroid function test

Management: *see page 54*

- T4 replacement therapy
- Monitoring of T4, TSH
- Monitoring of school performance, sleeping pattern and diet

Juvenile idiopathic arthritis (JIA)

- Age of onset is less than 16 years
- Duration of disease not less than 6 weeks
- Clinically: swelling, effusion, limitation of movement, pain and tenderness

	Systemic onset	Oligoarticular	Polyarticular RF -ve	Polyarticular RF +ve	Enthesitis
% from JIA	20%	40%	20%	10%	10%
Gender	M=F	F 80%	F 90%	F 80%	M 90%
Age	< 5 years	2-5 years	Any age	Late childhood	Late childhood
Joints	Polyarticular	Large joints; - Knee - Ankle - Wrist Tempro-mandibular joint	Symmetrical small and large joints	Symmetrical small and large joints	Large joints; - Hip - Sacroiliac - spine
Complications	-Fever 6 weeks -Salmon pink rash -HSM -↑LN -Anemia -Leukocytosis -Thrombocytopenia -Pericarditis -Weight loss	- Chronic uveitis - Leg length discrepancy			- Acute uveitis - Ankylosing spondylitis
ANA	-	+	+	+	-
RF	-	-	-	+	-

Management: *see page 54*

Specific:

- NSAIDs, injectional steroids, systemic steroids, methotrexate, infliximab
- Physiotherapy, occupational therapy, hydrotherapy, splints

Osteogenesis imperfecta

- It is a disorder of connective tissue
- Due to mutations of the genes encoding for type I collagen
- Type I collagen is found in bone, sclerae, ligaments

	I	**II**	**III**	**IV**
Inheritance	AD	AD / AR	AR	AD
Presentation	Osteoporosis Bone fragility Blue sclera Hearing loss	Osteoporosis Bone fragility	Osteoporosis Bone fragility Less blue	Osteoporosis Bone fragility Less blue
Prognosis	Spontaneous improvement with puberty	Lethal	Few survive to adolescence	Spontaneous improvement with puberty
X-Ray	Osteopenia Fractures	Osteopenia Fractures Fractures of ribs which is beaded and crumbled	Osteopenia Fractures	Osteopenia Fractures

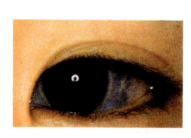
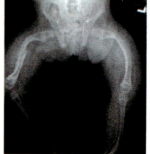
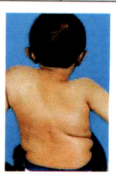

Management: *see page 54*

- Genetic counselling
- Careful nursing
- Splinting
- Correct deformities

Arthrogryposis syndromes

Main differential diagnosis is Osteogenesis imperfecta

Types:

Arthrogryposis multiplex congenita:

- Non-progressive
- Multiple joint contractures
- Normal facies, normal intelligence
- Hip dislocation, club foot

Distal Arthrogryposis

- Autosomal dominant
- Affects hands & feet

Larsen Syndrome

- Joints are affected but less rigid
- Multiple dislocations
- Scoliosis
- kyphosis

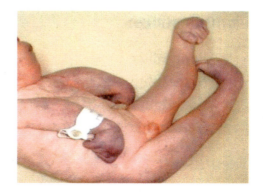

Kawasaki disease

- This is the most common acquired heart disease
- It is a multisystem disease that affects medium sized blood vessels
- Diagnosis depends on clinical picture

Criteria include fever more than 5 days + 4 out of the following 5 features

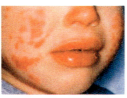 **Maculopapular rash** 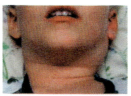 **Lymphadenopathy**

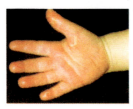 **Extremities changes** 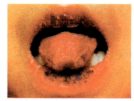 **Mucositis**

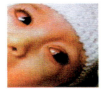 **Non purulent conjunctivitis**

Investigations:

CBC, ESR, CRP, anti-streptolysin O titer, viral studies, throat swab, ECG and Echocardiography

Complications:

- Pericarditis
- Myocarditis
- Endocarditis
- Coronary artery aneurisms

Treatment:

- High doses of IVIG / Aspirin

Henoch-Schonlein purpura

- This is inflammation of small vessels and capillaries
- More common in ages > 3 years
- More common in males than females

Pathophysiology:

May be due to precipitation of IgA complex in glomeruli and skin

Presentation:

- Skin
    - Petechial rash
    - Rash over lower limbs and buttocks
    - Cutaneous nodules
    - Subcutaneous edema
- Renal nephritis
- Arthritis
- Gastrointestinal bleeding and pain

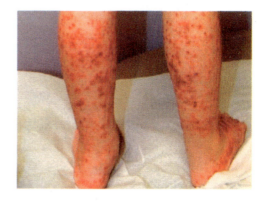

Investigations:

CBC, ESR, Urinalysis

Treatment:

Steroids in severe cases

Prognosis:

- Self-limiting
- Recurrence is common

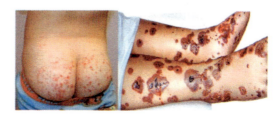

Perthes Disease

- Ischemic necrosis of femoral epiphysis of unknown etiology
- 4-9 years of age
- 15% are bilateral

C/P:
- Pain
- Limp
- Limitation of movement

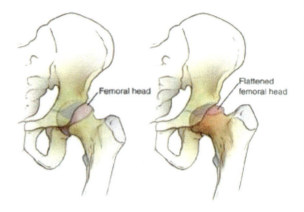

Stages:
1. Initial
2. Fragmentation
3. Healing
4. Residual

Differential diagnosis:
- Osteomyelitis
- Septic arthritis
- Synovitis
- Trauma
- Fracture
- Slipper upper femoral Capital epiphysis

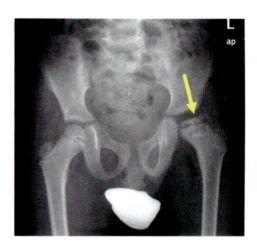

Investigation:

X-ray: Antero-Posterior, frog leg lateral

Management:
Decrease pain, stiffness and deformities by·
- Restriction of movement by non-operative bracing in abduction.
- Surgery in severe cases.

Psoriatic Arthritis

Don't Forget

"**Vancouver**" Criteria of diagnosis

Either:
- Arthritis + Psoriasis

Or

Arthritis + 3 out of 4 of the following;

- Dactylitis
- Onycholysis, nail pitting
- Psoriasis like rash
- Family history 1st, 2nd degree

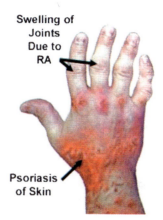

William's syndrome

- Abnormal deletion of chromosome 7 (FISH)
- Neonatal hypercalcemia
- Microcephaly
- IUGR
- Mild learning disability
- Cocktail Party Chatter
- Prominent lips
- Short palpebral fissures
- Stellate iris, blue eye
- Supravalvular aortic stenosis
- Peripheral pulmonary stenosis

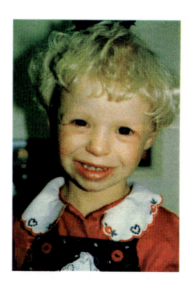

Beckwith – Weidemann syndrome

- It is a fetal overgrowth syndrome
- Most cases are sporadic

Criteria for diagnosis

3 major

2 major + 3 minor

Major	Minor
1. Overgrowth 2. Macroglossia 3. Abdominal wall defects	1. Ear lobe creases 2. Hemihypertrophy 3. Hypoglycemia 4. Organomegaly 5. Facial naevus

Presentation:

- **Infancy:**
    - Prematurity
    - Exomphalos
    - Hypoglycemia
- **Childhood:**
    - Macroglossia
        - Feeding problem
        - Speech problems
        - Obstructive apnea
    - Overgrowth more than 90th centile
    - Organomegaly
    - Hemihypertrophy
    - Risk of tumors
        - Wilms' tumor
        - Hepatoblastoma
        - Neuroblastoma

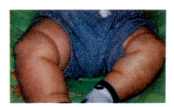
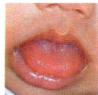
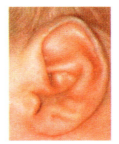
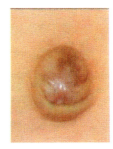

Immune disorders

X-Linked Agammaglobulinemia

- Defect in B cell development
- Mutation of Bruton tyrosine kinase gene

Presentation:

- Respiratory infection with streptococcus infection, influenza, mycoplasma
- Otitis media
- Sinusitis

Treatment: IVIG

IgA Deficiency:

- Most common primary immunodeficiency
- Respiratory, GI infection, atopy
- Associated with crohns' disease, ulcerative colitis, celiac disease and malignancy

Severe combined immunodeficiency:

- Defect in both cellular and humoral immunity
- X-linked or AR
- Males are more affected than females

Presentation:

- Severe recurrent Respiratory infection. RSV, CMV, PCP, adenovirus
- Diarrhea. Rota virus, adenovirus
- Skin rash

Management:

- Prophylactic (septrin, acyclovir, itraconazole)
- BMT
- Enzyme replacement; adenosine deaminase (ADA) and Gene therapy

CNS infection

Meningitis	Encephalitis
Neisseria meningitides B Streptococcal pneumonia HiB TB **Neonatal** Group B streptococcus, Listeria	Enterovirus Herpes Measles

Diagnosis: by lumbar puncture

Bacterial	:	↑ WBC, ↓↓ Glucose, ↑↑ Protein
Viral	:	↑ Lymphocytes
TB	:	↑ Lymphocytes
Partially treated bacteria	:	↑ Lymphocytes

Treatment:

Prophylaxis by vaccines (meningitis C, HiB)

1. < 3 months neonates : Ampicillin/cefotaxime
2. > 3 months child : 3rd generation; ceftriaxone
3. Viral or if unclear diagnosis : add acyclovir
4. If suspicious of TB : add anti-TB drugs
5. If overseas or multiple AB exposure : add vancomycin
6. Steroids. ↓ deafness, CNS defects in HiB

Complications:
- Sensori-neural deafness
- Convulsions
- Subdural collections

Bone infection

	Osteomyelitis	Septic Arthritis

Spread	- Hematogenous
	  ✓ Acute
	  ✓ Subacute
	  ✓ Chronic
	- Non-hematogenous
		Hematogenous

Site	Monoarticular Multiple	Monoarticular Multifocal in neonates
Organisms	**Neonate**: GBS, Staph, E.coli **Infant**: Strept, staph, Hib **Child**: Strept, staph, E. coli **SCA**: Strept, staph, salmonella	Strept, staph TB N meningitis N. Gonorrhea
Investigations	- ↑ WBC, ESR, CRP - Blood Culture - Needle Aspiration - X-ray - Bone Scan - MRI	same same US + aspiration CT scan
Treatment	4-6 weeks Antibiotics Surgery	2 weeks Antibiotics Surgical Drainage Needle aspiration

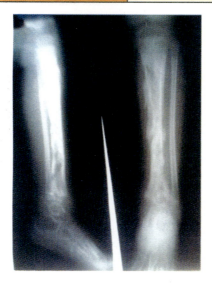

Osteomyelitis

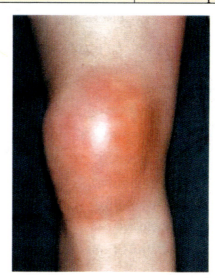

Septic arthritis

Tuberculosis

- Caused by Mycobacterium tuberculosis.
- Incubation period of 1 month.
- Children has primary disease.
- Children are rarely infectious.
- Children > Adults easily infected when exposed.

Types:

	TB Exposure	TB Infection	TB Disease
Maintenance	—	+	+
Clinically	—	—	+
C X R	—	—	+
Treat	No	Chemoprophylaxis	Chemotherapy

Pathogenesis:

Bacteria proliferate in the lung then → L.N

        Pulmonary macrophages ingest bacteria

      ↓ Cellular immune response

       → Ghon's focus

Clinical picture:
- Fever, cough
- Constitutional manifestation
- Miliary TB
- Meningitis
- Pericarditis
- Arthritis
- GI Infection

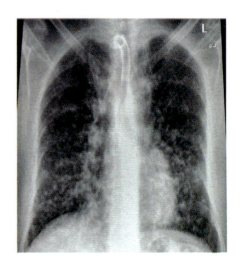

X-Ray Military TB

Diagnosis:

- Tuberculosis Test:
    - Heaf Test
    - Mantoux Test
        - Positive if induration area is 5 – 15 mm if no BCG given before.
- CXR
- PCR
- Zeil Nelsen stain of AFP from gastric wash, broncho-alveolar lavage
- Histology

Treatment:

Chemoprophylaxis	Chemotherapy
TB Infection	INH, Rifampicin for 6 months
Exposure of immunocompromised or HIV patients	Pyrazinamide + 4th drug for 1st 2 months
↓	Meningitis. treat for 12 months
INH for 6 months	
Or INH + Rifampicin for 3 months	

Neonatal contact with Tuberculosis Mother

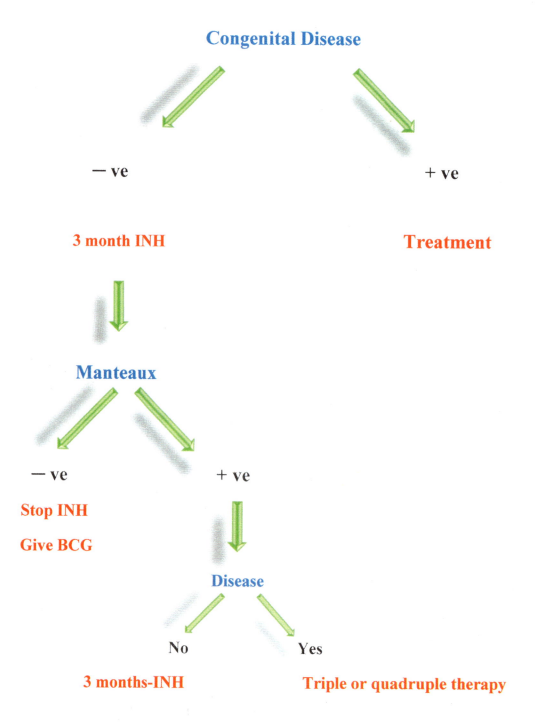

HIV

Transmission:

- Vertical
    - Prenatal
    - Intranatal
    - Postnatal
- Blood Product Transfusion
- Sexual transmission

Diagnosis:

- PCR viral detection
- Detection of IgG antibody to viral envelope protein

Presentation:

- Category N   Asymptomatic
- Category A   HSM, lymphadenopathy, Upper & lower RTI, otitis, sinusitis
- Category B   Pancytopenia, Meningitis, pneumonia, sepsis
- Category C
    - Severe bacterial infection
    - Candidiasis, cryptococcosis, coccidiomycosis
    - HIV, encephalopathy
    - Malignancy
    - PCP, herpes, CMV

Management:

- HAART
- PCP Prophylaxis
- Reduce vertical transmission by:
    - Caesarian section
    - HAART to mother and baby
    - No Breast Feeding

Infant of HIV mother

- Vertical transmission is the most common cause of childhood HIV
- One third across the placenta and two thirds during birth
- There is no associated embryopathy
- Babies are usually asymptomatic but later may show Hepatosplenomegaly and thrombocytopenia

Risk factors:

- Low maternal CD4 count
- High maternal viral load
- Presence of P24 antigen in the mother
- Preterm
- Premature rupture of membranes
- Vaginal birth
- No anti-retroviral treatment

Diagnosis:

1. HIV antibodies are positive at 18 months for 2 occasions
2. PCR is positive at any time for 2 occasions

Prophylaxis:

1. Anti-retroviral treatment to the mother in the 3rd trimester and to the baby 6 weeks postnatal
2. Avoidance of risk factors

This will decrease risk of transmission from 25% to 5%

Infants to HIV mother should receive:

- Early BCG vaccine
- Killed Salk vaccine

Herpes simplex virus

Types:
1. Skin, mucous membranes
2. Genital

Incubation   2-12 days

Transmission   direct contact

Presentation:
- Gingivostomatitis
- Keratoconjunctivitis
- Eczema herpeticum
- Meningoencephalitis
- Genital lesion
- Neonatal HSV

Diagnosis   PCR, electron microscopy

Treatment   Acyclovir IV, PO

Measles/Mumps/Rubella

	Measles	Mumps	Rubella
Incubation	1-2 weeks	2-3 weeks	2-3 weeks
Transmission	Respiratory	Respiratory	Respiratory Placental
Presentation	Prodrome of 3-5 days Fever, cough, conjunctival injection Koplik spots Eruptive Maculopapular rash	Fever Headache Painful parotids	Congenital Petichea Rash
Complication	Otitis media Bronchitis Pneumonia SSPE	Meningoencephalopathy Epididymitis Orchitis Pancreatitis	Encephalitis Arthritis
Treatment	Supportive		
Prophylaxis	MMR		

Malaria

- Caused by: Plasmodium (Vivax, Malarie, Ovale, Falciparum)
- Transmitted by: bite of female anopheles mosquito

Presentation:

- Fever, chills, rigors, sweating
- Nausea, vomiting, diarrhea
- Headache
- Pallor, jaundice
- HSM
- Malarie   Nephrotic syndrome
- Falciparum.
  - ✓ Cerebral malaria
  - ✓ Anemia
  - ✓ Hypoglycemia
  - ✓ Renal Failure
  - ✓ Pulmonary edema

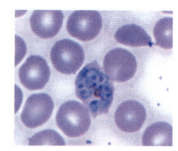

Diagnosis   thick, thin blood film

Treatment:

- **Vivax, ovale**:   Chloroquine
  Primaquine → ↓ hepatic stage
- **Malarie**:   Chloroquine
- **Falciparum**:   Quinine
  Fansidar: Consider at last day of quinine therapy

Prophylaxis:

- Protective clothing
- Bed net
- Mosquito repellent

Typhoid fever

Organism Salmonella typhi, paratyphi
Transmission Faeco-oral route
Presentation:
- Fever
- Headache
- Constipation, diarrhea, abdominal pain
- HSM
- Rose spots

Complication:
- Intestinal perforation
- Severe hemorrhage
- Osteomyelitis, meningitis

Investigation: Blood, stool, BMA cultures

Treatment: Ampicillin/ ceftriaxone/cefotaxime/chloramphenicol

Leishmaniasis

Types:

- Cutaneous   ulcers at exposed skin
- Mucosal   oral, nasopharyngeal lesions
- Visceral   HSM, Pancytopenia, LN↑

Diagnosis   Microscopic detection of intracellular parasites

Treatment:
- Amphotericin B
- Na Stibogluconate

Congenital infections

Presentation:

1. Sensorineural Hearing Loss
2. Microcephaly
3. Cataracts
4. Chorioretinitis
5. HSM
6. Petichea
7. Pneumonitis

CMV   calcification (periventricular)

Rubella   microphthalmia, cardiac disorders, bony lesion

Toxoplasma hydrocephalus, calcification (diffuse)

Diagnosis:

- TORCH
- PCR
- Ophthalmology examination

Treatment:

- Vaccination (Rubella)
- Spiramycin (Toxoplasma)
- Ganciclovir (CMV)

Lung function tests

- **FVC**: total amount of air exhaled during forced expiration
- **FEV1**: total amount of air exhaled in 1st second
- **PEFR**: The highest forced expiratory flow measured with a peak flow meter
- **FEFx**: Forced expiratory flow related to some portion of the FVC curve; modifiers refer to amount of FVC already exhaled

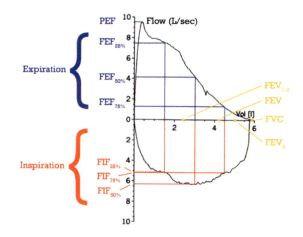

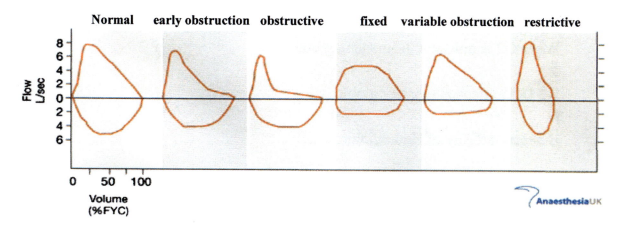

Lung volumes

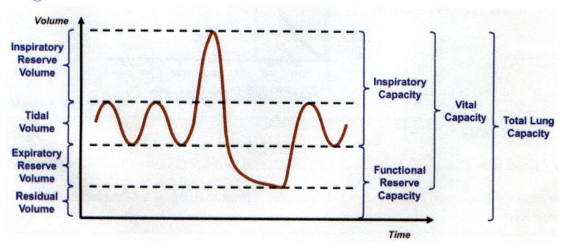

Oxygen dissociation curve

Hemoglobin Molecule

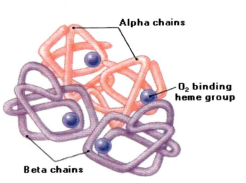

4 subunits
↓
Each unit
↙ ↘
Globin   Hemo
↓
α or B

- Fe combines to O_2
- Hb molecule attach 4 O_2

Adult Hb 2 α + 2 B

When O2 is unloaded from Hemoglobin
↓
2-3 DPG attached to Hemoglobin
↓
Decrease affinity of Hemoglobin to O2

↑ O_2 Affinity

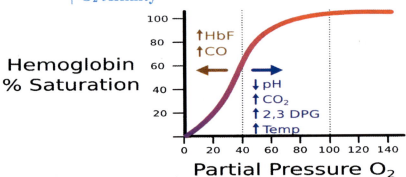

↓ O2 Affinity

Bohr Effect:

Lung: Alveoli takes CO_2 - ↓ CO_2 in blood - ↑ PH in blood   Shift to Left → ↑ O2 Affinity of blood

Tissue: Gets off CO_2 - ↑ CO_2 in blood - ↓ PH in blood   Shift to Right → ↓ O2 Affinity of blood leaving it at tissue level

Sore throat

Centor score

1. Tonsiller exudate
2. Tender cervical nodes
3. Fever
4. No cough

The higher the score the higher the risk of infection with streptococcus

- Routine throat swab (not indicated)
- Analgesics are all what is required unless severe cases
- Penicillin or macrolide are preferred antibiotics
- Co-amoxiclave should be avoided

Tonsillectomy

Indication:

- Severe and disabling disease
- 7 times tonsillitis a year
- 5 times tonsillitis every year for 2 years
- 3 times tonsillitis every year for 3 years

Post-operative nausea/vomiting

- Dexamethasone
- NSAID
- Antiemetics

Bronchiolitis

- Common in the first 3-6 months of birth
- Commonest in winter
- Due to infection with Respiratory syncytial virus (RSV)

Presentation:

- Cough + nasal discharge + inspiratory crackle + expiratory wheeze
- Signs of respiratory distress

Risk Factors:

- Prematurity
- CHD
- CLD
- Smoking
- Immunodeficiency

Breast feeding decreases the Risk of Bronchiolitis

Investigation:

- Pulse oximeter
- Rapid testing for RSV

In disease uncertainty do:
- CXR
- CBC, electrolytes
- Arterial blood gases

Treatment:

- Saline drops, suction, O2 (humidified), NG feeding, good hydration
- Palivizumab Prophylaxis. if <1 year / CHD / CLD / Immunodeficiency / Prematurity

Indication for Admission:

Cyanosis, RR> 70/min, Poor feeding, apnea, lethargy, O2 saturation < 94%

Asthma

- Affects 10% of preschool
- 30% of school age

Clinical Features:
1. Wheezes, cough, difficult breathing, chest tightness
2. Worse at night, early morning
3. Worse with exercise & other triggers
4. History of atopic disorder
5. Family history of asthma, or atopy
6. Improvement with adequate therapy

After Assessment ➡ probability of Asthma

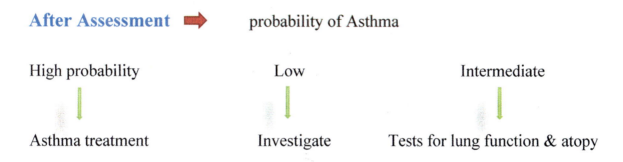

High probability	Low	Intermediate
Asthma treatment	Investigate	Tests for lung function & atopy

Non pharmacological Management:
1. Breast feeding
2. Avoidance of smoking
3. Weight reduction
4. Prevent house dust mites
5. Regular exercise
6. Peak flow diary

Other precautions with insufficient evidence:
- Allergen avoidance
- Immunotherapy
- Pet avoidance
- Acupuncture
- Herbal & Chinese medicine

Pharmacologic Management of Asthma

Aim:
1. No daytime symptoms
2. No night time awakening
3. No need for rescue medication
4. No exacerbation
5. No limitation of activity
6. Normal lung functions

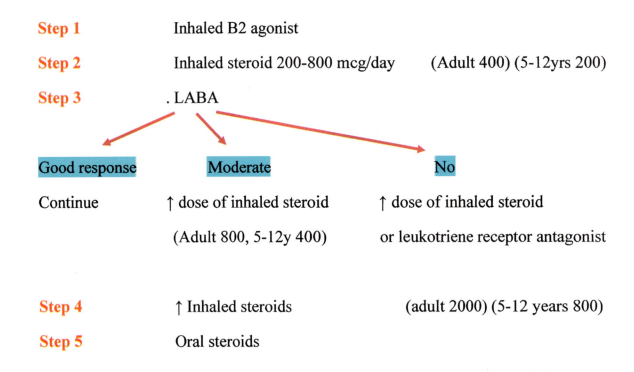

Step 1	Inhaled B2 agonist
Step 2	Inhaled steroid 200-800 mcg/day (Adult 400) (5-12yrs 200)
Step 3	. LABA

| Good response | Moderate | No |
| Continue | ↑ dose of inhaled steroid (Adult 800, 5-12y 400) | ↑ dose of inhaled steroid or leukotriene receptor antagonist |

| Step 4 | ↑ Inhaled steroids (adult 2000) (5-12 years 800) |
| Step 5 | Oral steroids |

Children < 5 years

Step 1	B2 agonist
Step 2	Inhaled steroids 200-400 mcg/day
Step 3	Leukotriene receptor antagonist
Step 4	Refer to specialist

Acute & Life Threatening Asthma

Acute	Life Threatening
PEF 33-50% of best	PEF < 33%
RR > 25/min	PO2 < 92%
HR > 110/min	Silent chest
Inability to complete sentence	Cyanosis
	Arrhythmia
	Exhaustion
	Altered conscious

Management:

1. O2 supply to keep saturation > 94%
2. B2 agonist inhalation (nebulizer)
3. Steroid therapy & continue 5 days
4. Nebulized Ipratropium bromide.
5. IV MgSO4 for asthma with no response
6. IV aminophylline only in PICU for unresponsive cases

Reasons for poor response to Asthma treatment:

1. Poor compliance
2. Poor inhaler's technique
3. Poor understanding of the disease and management
4. Environmental, triggering factors
5. Stress, physical, psychological factors
6. Wrong diagnosis

Inhaler devices

- Drug delivery by inhalation is superior to oral intake
- There is no difference between devices if used correctly

Can be either:

MDI (metered dose inhalers)	DPI (dry powder inhalers) or breath activated inhalers
Depends on hand to lung coordination	Depends on inspiratory forces

Uses of spacer: large volume or small volume spacers
1. Children of any age, and with a mask if less than 2 years
2. Adult with poor coordination
3. In acute asthma attack
4. Should be cleaned monthly, washed with warm water and left to dry in air to avoid electrostatic charges interfere with the drug
5. Should be replaced every 12 months

Types and technique:

Type	Image	Age
MDI ✓ Shake ✓ 1 puff ✓ 1 breath ✓ Hold breath for 10 seconds	MDI Inhaler	Any age
MDI with spacer ✓ Shake ✓ 1 puff ✓ 4 breaths in and out		Preferred below 5 years With mask before 2 years
Accuhaler ✓ Rotate ✓ Activate ✓ 1 deep breath ✓ Hold breath for 10 seconds	Accuhaler	Above 8 years
Turbohaler ✓ Rotate right and left ✓ 1 deep breath ✓ Hold breath for 10 seconds	Turbohaler	
Autohalar ✓ Shake ✓ Activate ✓ 1 deep breath ✓ Hold breath for 10 seconds		

After user of preventer devises don't forget to **RINSE, GARGLE, SPIT** to avoid local complication of steroids (sore throat, oropharyngeal thrush, hoarseness of voice)

Bronchiectasis

- Chronically inflamed and dilated airways
- Most common in the lower lobes of both lungs followed by middle lobes

Triad of:

- Airways obstruction
- Retained secretions
- Infection

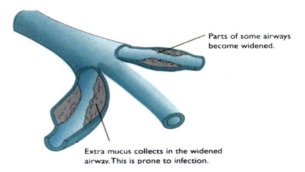

Causes:

Infectious:

- ✓ Staphylococcal, streptococcal, pertussis and influenza infection
- ✓ Immunodeficiency; IgA deficiency, Job's syndrome, complement deficiency
- ✓ Primary ciliary dyskinesia

Obstruction:

- ✓ Asthma
- ✓ Bronchiolitis obliterans
- ✓ Lobar sequestration
- ✓ Lymphadenopathy and tumors

Retained secretions:

- ✓ Recurrent aspiration

Management: *see page 54*

1. Infection — prophylactic antibiotics
2. Obstruction — bronchodilators
3. Retained secretions — mucolytic
4. Surgery, lobectomy in severe cases
5. Physiotherapy for life
6. Monitoring: spirometry, sputum cultures, monitor growth and nutrition

Chronic lung disease

- Requirement of respiratory support with or without ventilation after birth
- Oxygen dependency at 28 days
- Evidence of respiratory distress and chest X-Ray changes

Risk factors:

- **B**arotrauma
- **P**rolonged & high levels of inspired oxygen
- **P**rematurity
- **P**DA
- **P**rolonged ventilation
- **P**ulmonary infection
- **P**neumothorax

Presentation:

- Small for age
- Hyper-expanded chest
- Respiratory distress
- Stridor, wheezes
- Others: scaphocephaly, chest drains, PDA, gastrostomy

Differential diagnosis:

- Congenital heart disease
- Bronchiectasis
- Immunodeficiency

Management:

1. Oxygen supplementation
2. Maintain good nutrition
3. Steroids to decrease O2 requirement
4. Diuretics to improve lung function
5. Physiotherapy
6. Vaccination with influenza, palivizumab

Kyphoscoliosis

This is a lateral curvature of the spine with rotation of vertebral bodies

Types:

- ✓ Positional — corrected with bending down
- ✓ Structural — doesn't correct

Causes:

- Cerebral palsy
- Duchenne muscular dystrophy
- Spinal muscle atrophy
- Friedreich's ataxia
- Marfan syndrome
- Homocystinuria
- Mucopolysaccharidosis
- Osteogenesis imperfecta

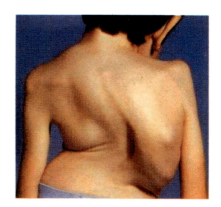

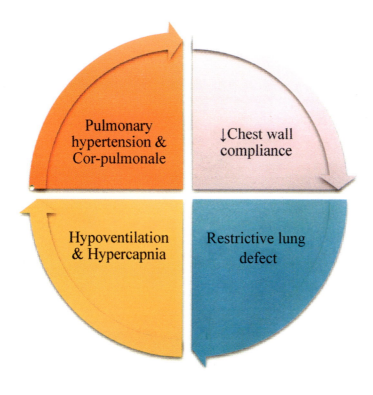

Investigation:

- Chest X-Ray
- Lung functions
- O2 saturation monitoring

Treatment:

- Corrective orthopedic surgery

Stridor

Types:

- **Inspiratory** : extra-thoracic obstruction
- **Biphasic** : obstruction at the level of glottis, subglottis and trachea
- **Expiratory** : intra-thoracic obstruction

Causes:

- Sick child
    1. Epiglottitis
    2. Bacterial tracheitis
    3. Inhaled foreign body
    4. Anaphylaxis
    5. Hypocalcemia
- Not sick child
    1. Laryngomalacia
    2. Tracheomalacia
    3. Bronchomalacia
    4. Tracheal web
    5. Tracheal hemangioma
    6. Vascular ring
    7. Tumors

Investigations

- Serum calcium level
- Chest X-Ray
- Bronchoscopy
- Rigid laryngoscopy
- Barium swallow
- Trans-esophageal Echo
- Lung function test

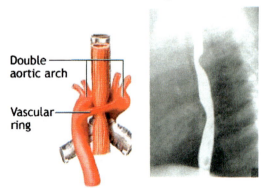

Vascular ring

Chronic fatigue syndrome

- F: M = 3:1
- 50-100/100000 population
- Characterized by Physical & mental disability

Presentation:

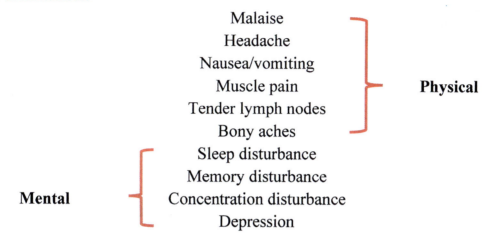

Physical:
- Malaise
- Headache
- Nausea/vomiting
- Muscle pain
- Tender lymph nodes
- Bony aches

Mental:
- Sleep disturbance
- Memory disturbance
- Concentration disturbance
- Depression

Diagnosis:
- History & physical examination
- Exclude other clinical causes

Investigation:
- CBC, blood film, electrolytes, liver enzymes
- ESR
- Random blood sugar
- CK, Thyroid function
- Urine analysis

Management: *see page 54*
- Lifestyle (dieting advice, sleep problems, graded exercise)
- Monitoring (school, growth)
- Referrals (psychology, occupational, physiotherapy)
- Symptom treatment:
    - Pain
    - Depression

Coagulation pathways

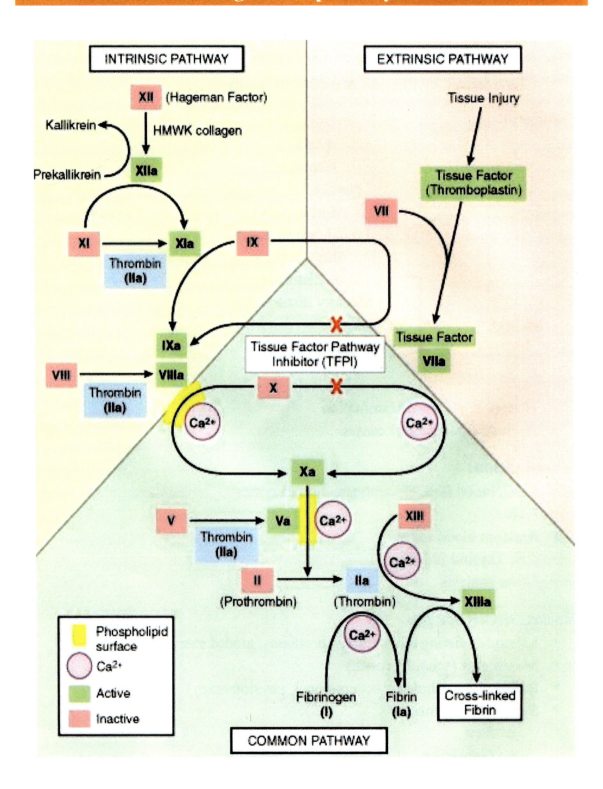

Constipation

Most important to exclude:

1. Hypothyroidism
2. Hirschsprung disease
3. DIOS
4. Spina bifida

Importance points in history & examination:

1. Stool pattern. hard, soft, frequency/week
2. Timing + Precipitation factors. changing in diet, housing, school, potty training
3. Defecation. pain, strain, blood
4. History·
   - Previous constipation
   - Previous anal fissure
5. Thyroid status
6. Meconium passage
7. Lower limb symptoms
8. Growth
9. Diet, fluid intake

Examination: neurologic, abdomen, back, perianal area

Management:

Dis-impaction	Maintenance
Polyethylene glycol (escalating dose) If not tolerated or no effect 2 weeks ↓ - Stimulant laxative (senna or Docusate Na) - Osmotic laxative (lactulose)	Polyethylene glycol Stimulant or osmotic laxatives (if not tolerated) - Maintain for several weeks - Stop gradually

Cerebral Palsy

- Persistent disorders of movement, posture and tone due to non-progressive defects in the developing immature brain

Specific features

Causes

Prenatal	Natal	Postnatal
Prematurity Chromosomal anomalies Cerebral malformation Infections Maternal alcohol and substance abuse	HIE Intracranial hemorrhage Kernicterus Hypoglycemia	Trauma Infection Stroke Intracranial hemorrhage

Complications

- Spasticity and contractures
- Musculoskeletal like scoliosis
- Pseudo bulbar palsy, feeding problems and GI reflux
- Speech problems
- Learning difficulties
- Developmental delay
- Social impact

Clinical picture

Hemiplegic/diplegic	Quadriplegic	Ataxic	Athetoid
1. Weakness is more distally 2. In diplegia: legs > arms	1. All 4 limbs are affected 2. First hypotonic then spastic 3. Bulbar muscles affected	1. Cerebral ataxia 2. With diplegia	1. Abnormal involuntary movement 2. Lesion in extrapyramidal system or basal ganglia 3. Kernicterus, HIE

Investigations

Indication:
1. No obvious cause
2. Loss of skills
3. Lower motor neuron lesions
4. Symmetrical lesions
5. Unusual symptoms (ataxia, nystagmus)

Investigations:
1. CT, MRI brain
2. MRI spine
3. Chromosomal analysis
4. EEG
5. Infectious screening
6. Metabolic screening
7. Ophthalmologic assessment
8. Hearing assessment

Management

1. Family education
2. Life style
3. Contact group and organizations
4. Helping with DLA, SEN
5. Monitoring of growth, development

Referrals:
- General pediatrics: coordinator
- Physiotherapist: prevention and treatment of contractures
- Occupational therapist: modify the environment according to child's requirements
- Speech therapist
- Dietitian
- Orthopedic surgeon
- Health educator
- Social worker

	Crohn's disease	Coeliac disease
Specific Feature	• 5:100000 of under 16 years of age • Uveitis or episcleritis • Arthritis • Erythema nodosum, pyoderma gangrenosum, erythema multiforme • Growth failure • Delayed bone maturation • Delayed sexual maturation	• Prevalence of 2% in western Europe • Dermatitis herpetiform • Iron deficiency anemia • Short stature • Autoimmune thyroid disease • Mixed connective tissue disease • Pernicious anemia. Diabetes mellitus
Pathophysiology	• Chronic inflammatory disorder involving any region of the bowel from mouth to anus • Inflammation is transmural, with skip lesions • Mucosa is granulomatous with deep ulcers	• Gluten sensitive enteropathy with intolerance to gluten present in BOWR (barley, Oat, Wheat, Rye)
Clinical picture	• Abdominal pain • Diarrhea • Weight loss • Systemic upset and fever, lethargy	• After 6 months of age • Chronic diarrhea • Weight loss • Abdominal distension, Lethargy / irritability
Investigations	• Raised inflammatory markers • Upper GI endoscope and biopsy • Barium study to determine the extent	• Diagnosis Duodenal or jejunum biopsy showing: ✓ Sub-total villous atrophy ✓ Crypt hypertrophy ✓ Intra-epithelial lymphocytes ✓ Lamina propria plasma cell infiltrate • Screening Tissue transglutaminase(tTG) with serum IgA

Treat	A. Family education
	B. Contact groups and organizations
	C. Monitoring of growth and side effects of medications
	D. Referrals: dietician, surgeon
	E. Specific:
	  1. Exclusive enteral feeding (elemental or polymeric diet) for 8 weeks ➔ remission in 80% of patients
	  2. Anti-inflammatory (ASA)
	  3. Steroids in severe disease and relapses
	  4. Azathioprine and anti TNF monoclonal antibodies in refractory disease
	  5. Antibiotics for abscesses
	  6. Surgery for:
	    a) Persistent symptoms
	    b) Intolerable side effects
	    c) Abscesses
	    d) Toxic megacolon
		A. Family education
		B. Contact groups and organizations
		C. Monitoring of growth and increased incidence of bowel cancers
		D. Referrals: dietician
		E. Specific:
		  Gluten free diet for life
		
		Indication for gluten challenge:
		✓ Diagnostic uncertainty
		✓ Diagnosis before 2 years of age due to presence of other causes that lead to villous atrophy

Cystic Fibrosis

Specific features
- AR
- Prevalence: 1:2500
- Carrier frequency: 1:25

Pathophysiology
- Defect in CF transmembrane regulator gene leads to defective secretion of chloride, Na, water results in viscid secretions
- Most common mutation = Delta F508

Clinical picture

Respiratory
1. Bacterial colonization and infection
2. Allergic Bronchopulmonary aspergellosis (wheezes, high IgE, eosinophilia, +ve culture for Aspergellosis)
3. Asthma
4. Corpulmonale (HM, edema, raised JVP)

GIT
1. Malabsorption
2. Meconium ileus
3. DIOS (abdominal pain and mass)
4. Rectal prolapse
5. Obstructive jaundice
6. Liver fibrosis
7. Biliary cirrhosis & portal hypertension

Endocrine
1. Pancreatic insufficiency
2. IDDM
3. Impaired glucose tolerance
4. Pancreatitis

Others
- Hyponatremia
- Hypochloremic metabolic alkalosis
- Infertility

Investigations
- Antenatal: chorionic villous sampling, amniocentesis
- Immunoreactive trypsin (IRT)
- Genetic analysis
- Sweat test
  - Pilocarpine iontophoresis
  - 100 mg of sweat required
  - Test over 30 minutes
  - Sweat chloride >60 mmol/l is diagnostic
  - Unreliable in dehydration, rash, edema, on steroids

Management

1. **Physiotherapy**
   - Percussion, vibration & gravity
   - PEP, coughing
   - Regular exercise program
2. **Nutrition**
   - Monitor of growth
   - High calories and high protein
   - Vitamin (ADEK)
   - NGT, Gastrostomy
3. **Pancreatic enzymes**
4. **Antibiotics**
   - Colonization by Staph and pseudomonas treated by Flucloxacillin and Nebulized tobramycin, colomycin
   - Acute infection treated by oral Cipro or IV ceftazidime/gentamycin
   - Infection with Burkolderia Cepacia treated with Meropenem
5. **DNase**
   - Digest viscous secretions
6. **Separation of patient**
7. **Gene therapy**
8. **Treatment of complication**
   - Asthma
   - ABPA: steroids
   - Corpulmonale: heart lung transplant
   - Diabetes: insulin
   - DIOS: laxatives / surgery
   - Arthritis
   - Liver disease: ursodeoxycholic acid

Nephrotic syndrome

Specific features

- Abnormalities with the kidney leading to leakage of protein ...... Triad of :
1. Hypoalbuminemia: albumin < 25 gm/dl
2. Proteinuria: protein/creatinine > 200 mg/mmol
3. Edema

Complications & treatment

- **Infection**
  - Due to loss of immunoglobulins, complement, edema
  - Mostly due to pneumococcus and haemophilus influenza
  - Vulnerable to chicken pox and measles
  - Peritonitis

  ⬆
  - Prophylactic penicillin
  - Vaccination : pneumococcal, influenza
  - IV antibiotics

- **Hypovolemia**
  - Tachycardia
  - Tachypnea
  - Wide pulse pressure
  - Prolonged capillary refill
  - Decreased urine output

  ⬆
  - IV fluids and Fluid balance
  - Dietician: low salt, normal protein
  - Albumin and Lasix

- **Thrombosis**
  - Due to loss of protein C and S. loss of antithrombin III
  - Immobilization

  ⬆
  - Mobilization
  - Adequate hydration

- **Hypertension**
- **Acute and chronic renal failure**

Clinical picture

1. Puffy eye lids
2. Lower limb edema
3. Ascites
4. Pleural pericardial effusion
5. Scrotal, vulvar edema
6. Tachypnea & tachycardia
7. Pallor

Investigations:

1. CBC, electrolytes, LFTs, ESR, CRP
2. Albumin, C3, C4
3. Urinalysis, dipstick
4. ANA, Anti DS DNA antibodies
5. Anti streptolysin O titer

Indication of renal biopsy
1. Age <1 or >12 years
2. Hypertension
3. Hematuria
4. Renal failure
5. Steroid resistance, Steroid dependent, Frequent relapses

6. Referrals:
- General pediatrics
- Nephrologist
- Dietitian
- Health educator
- Social worker

Recommended urine dipstick
1. Daily till remission
2. Twice weekly in tapering
3. Daily if unwell

Management

1. Family education
2. Life style (diet, exercise)
3. Contact group and organizations
4. Monitoring of growth, development, fluid
5. Steroid therapy: prednisolone 60 mg/m2 for 28 days followed by 40 mg/m2 alternate days

	VSD	ASD	AVSD	AR	PS	AS
Specific Feature	• 30% of CHD • Membranous part	• 7% of CHD • Most common is ostium secondum	• 5% of CHD • Down syndrome (30% of CHD in Down)	• 5% of CHD • Turner, Marfan, Ehler Danlos	• 5% of CHD • Sub V, valvular, supra V • Noonan, Williams	• 5% of CHD • Sub V, valvular, supra V, subaortic • Turner, William
Pathphysiology	• Left to right shunt • Left vent. Volume overload • Increased pulmonary blood flow	• Left to right shunt • Right vent. Volume overload • Increased pulmonary blood flow	• Left to right shunt • Rt, Lt vent. Volume overload • Increased pulmonary blood flow	Left vent. Volume overload	Right vent. Pressure overload	Left vent. Pressure overload
Sympt.	• Small defect: asymptomatic • Large defect: Heart failure	Mostly asymptomatic	• Small defect: asymptomatic • Large defect: Heart F.	• Reduced exercise tolerance • Risk of ischemia	• Usually no symptoms • Cyanosis if severe	• Mostly no symptoms • Chest pain, syncope
Examin	Is it hemodynamically significant? • Effect on growth • Tachypnea • Displaced apex • Loud S2 • Soft murmur - Normal S1 S2, loud S2 if PH - Pansystolic murmur LLSE	- Wide Fixed splitting of S2 - Ejection systolic murmur over ULSE	Is it hemodynamically significant? • Effect on growth • Tachypnea • Displaced apex - Pansystolic murmur LLSE heard - mitral regurge murmur	• Water hammer pulse • Collapsing carotid pulse • Wide pulse pressure • Thrill at LSE • Diastolic murmur at LSE increase by leaning and expiration	• Thrill at ULSE • Ejection systolic murmur at ULSE, to back	• Thrill at URSE, suprasternal, carotid • Ejection systolic murmur at URSE, to neck
CXR	Increased vascular markings Cardiomegaly	Increased vasc. markings Cardiomegaly	Increased vasc. markings Cardiomegaly	Cardiomegaly	Cardiomegaly	Cardiomegaly
ECG	Cardiomegaly (left vent)	• Cardiomegaly (right vent) • Partial RBBB • Axis deviation	• Cardiomegaly (right vent) • Superior axis	Cardiomegaly (left vent)	Cardiomegaly (right vent)	Cardiomegaly (left vent)
ECHO	Diagnostic					
Treat	Small: watch and wait Large: anti HF measures • Diuretics • Captopril • High calories Surgical closure when ratio between pulm:syst blood flow > 2:1 • 6 months if significant • 2-5 years if moderate	Closure at 3-5 years by: • Trans-catheter device • surgery	anti HF measures • Diuretics • Captopril • High calories Surgical closure at 4-6 months	Valve replacement in exercise induced symptoms Anticoagulant post repair	Surgery depends on pressure gradient across stenotic valve	Surgery depends on pressure gradient across stenotic valve

	COA	Fallot's Tetralogy
Specific Feature	• 5% of CHD • Juxtaductal=most common • Preductal=severe, presents in neonates • Turner, bicuspid aortic valve	• 5% of CHD • Most common cyanotic HD • 25% associated with right side aortic arch
Pathphysiology		• Right ventricular hypertrophy • Pulmonary stenosis • Overriding aorta • VSD

Sympt.	Disparities in pulse and BP in upper and lower limbs	• Arrhythmia
		• Brain abscess
		• Cerebral thrombosis
		• Cyanotic spills
		   - Knee chest position
		   - Morphine
		   - Na bicarb.
		   - B-blockers
		   - vasoconstrictors
		• **Dyspnea**
		• **Endocarditis**

Examln.	• BP in lower limb < upper limb • Weak femoral pulses • Radio-femoral delay • Ejection systolic murmur at the interscapular area After surgery: • Left lateral thoracotomy • Absent left radial pulse	• Central cyanosis • Clubbing • Absent pulse at side of BT shunt • Scars: lateral or median • Thrill over ULSE • Ejection systolic murmur at ULSE transmitting through lungs
CXR	• Cardiomegaly(left) if severe • Rib notching	• Boot shaped heart (right vent hypertrophy) • Pulmonary oligaemia
ECG	Cardiomegaly(left) if severe	• Cardiomegaly • Right axis deviation
	Diagnostic	
Treat	Subclavian flab or end to end anastomosis	BT shunt followed by definitive repair at 4-12 months depending on: • Severity • Type of anatomy • Size of child

ECG

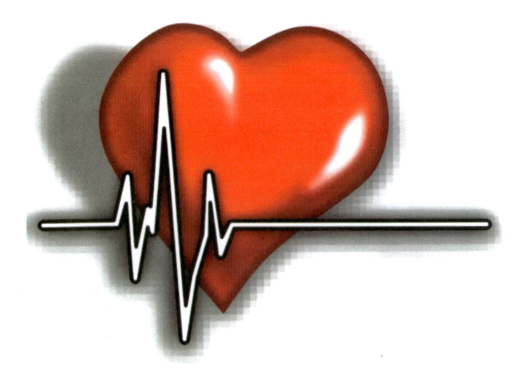

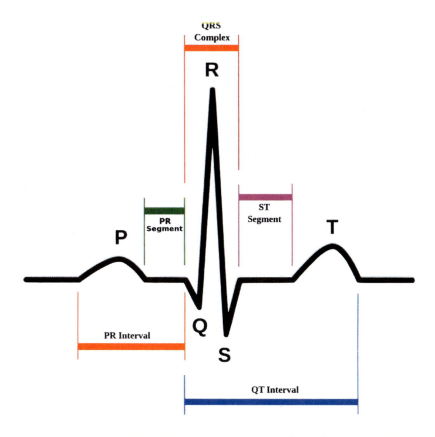

Sinus rhythm

1. P wave before each QRS
2. Regular PR interval
3. At least upright in I, aVF and inverted in aVR and usually upright in II

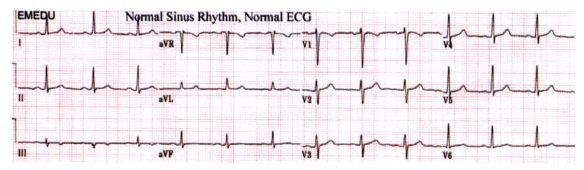

Heart rate

300 / number of large square between RR intervals

Sinus tachycardia

Heart rate is > 140-160 bpm in children and infants respectively

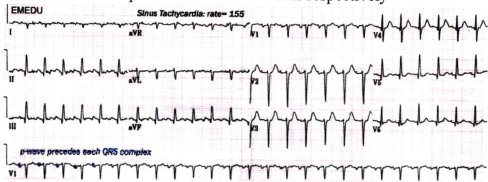

Sinus bradycardia

Heart rate is < 60-70 bpm in children and older children respectively

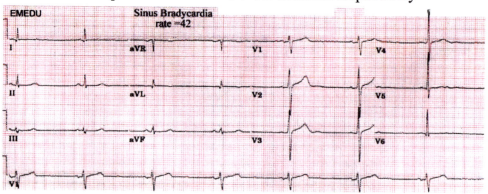

Sinus arrhythmia

Normal P-QRS configuration, but irregular heart rate which increases during inspiration and decreases during expiration.

Sick sinus syndrome

- Occurs mainly after surgery of the atria or the atrial septum
- May occur as sinus bradycardia, sinus arrest, and paroxysmal atrial tachycardia.
- If symptomatic it will need pacemaker insertion.

Axis determination

I	aVF	Axis
+	+	Left
+	-	Left
-	+	Right
-	-	Right

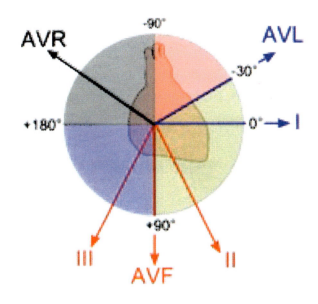

Right axis deviation	Left axis deviation	Superior axis
Right ventricular hypertrophy RBBB	Left ventricular hypertrophy LBBB Left anterior hemiblock	Tricuspid atresia Epstein's anomaly Noonan's syndrome W-P-W syndrome AVSD Left anterior hemiblock

PR interval

Normal: 0.12-0.2 sec

Prolonged PR interval:

1. Myocarditis
2. Rheumatic fever
3. Ischemia
4. Hyperkalemia
5. Digitalis, Digoxin toxicity
6. Hypothermia
7. Duchenne muscular atrophy

Short PR interval:

1. Cardiomyopathies
2. Pomp's disease
3. Fredreich's ataxia
4. W-P-W
5. Duchenne muscular dystrophy

QRS complex

Normal: 0.05-0.08 sec

Wide QRS:

1. BBB
2. W-P-W
3. Arrhythmia of ventricular origin
4. Intraventricular block
5. Ventricular hypertrophy

QRS amplitude

High voltage	Low voltage
1. Ventricular hypertrophy 2. BBB 3. WBW 4. Intraventricular block	1. Myocarditis 2. Pericardial effusion 3. Constrictive pericarditis 4. Thick chest wall

Q wave

Normal amplitude: < 5mm
Normal duration: 0.02-0.03 sec

No Q wave in V6:
1. Dextrocardia
2. Transposition of great arteries
3. Single ventricle
4. LBBB

Q wave in V1:
1. RVH
2. Transposition of great arteries
3. Single ventricle

Deep Q wave:
1. LVH, RVH
2. Biventricular hypertrophy
3. Cardiomyopathy

Deep and wide Q wave:
1. Myocardial infarction
2. Myocardial fibrosis

Abnormal T wave

Tall peaked T wave:

1. Hyperkalemia
2. LVH
3. Posterior myocardial infarction

Flat or low T wave

1. Hypokalemia
2. Hypothyroidism
3. Pericarditis
4. Myocarditis
5. Ischemia
6. Hypo / hyperglycemia

Long QT syndromes

Prolonged QT:
1. Jervell-lange-nelson syndrome (AR with deafness)
2. Romano-ward syndrome (AD non-lethal)
3. Hypocalcaemia, hypokalemia, hypomagnesaemia, hypothermia
4. Myocarditis
5. WBW
6. BBB
7. Head injuries and CVA
8. Drugs:
   - Erythromycin
   - TMP
   - TCAs
   - Antiarrhythmic
   - Cisapride
   - Methadone

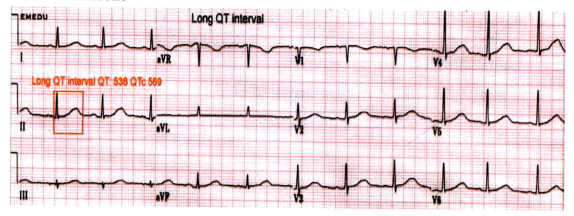

Premature atrial contraction (PAC)

The beat is premature occurring before the next cycle is due.
High : P wave is upright in II
Low : P wave is negative in II

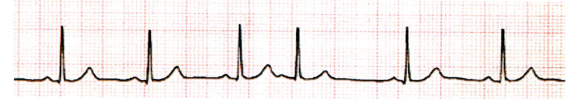

Atrial hypertrophy

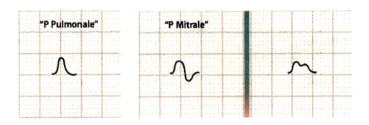

P Pulmonale: Right atrial hypertrophy

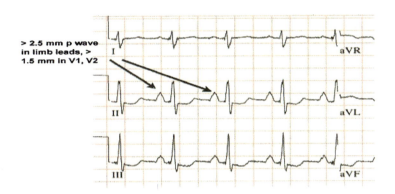

> 2.5 mm p wave in limb leads, > 1.5 mm in V1, V2

P Mitrale: Left atrial hypertrophy

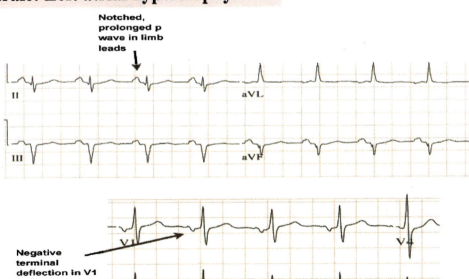

Notched, prolonged p wave in limb leads

Negative terminal deflection in V1

Right ventricular hypertrophy

1. Right axis deviation
2. R in V1, V2   large   R/S high
3. S in I, V6   large   R/S low
4. T wave upright in V1
5. Q wave in V1

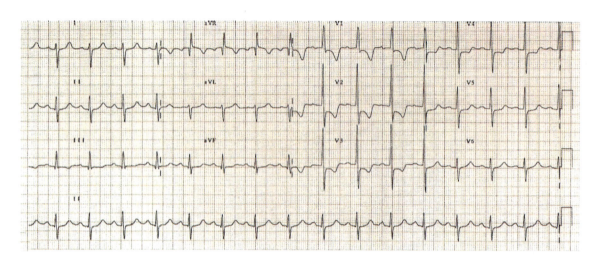

Left ventricular hypertrophy

1. Left axis deviation
2. R in V5, V6, I, II, III   large   R/S low
3. S in V1, V2   large   R/S high

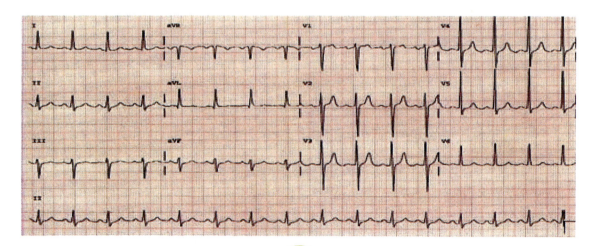

Right bundle branch block RBBB

1. Open heart surgery
2. ASD
3. Coarctation
4. Epstein's anomaly
5. Cardiomyopathy
6. Duchenne muscle dystrophy
7. Myotonic dystrophy
8. Kearn's sayre syndrome

Criteria:

1. Right axis deviation
2. Wide QRS
3. **MarroW**   M = RSR   in V1, V2
                       W= R with slurred **s**   in V5, V6

Left bundle branch block LBBB

1. Ischemic heart disease
2. Hypertrophic cardiomyopathy
3. Surgery of left ventricle

Criteria:

1. Left axis deviation
2. Wide QRS
3. **WillaM**   W= wide **s**   in V1, V2
                       M= RSR   in I, V5, V6

4. No Q wave in V5, V6

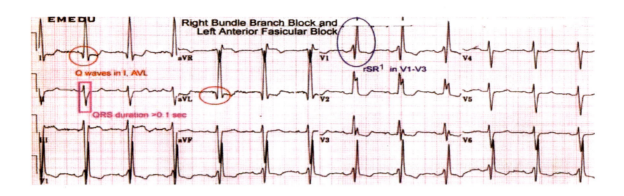

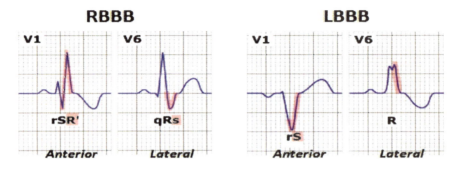

Pre-excitation =WPW= (AV) reentry tachycardia

Excitation of the ventricle through a pathway other than the normal way

Criteria:
1. Short PR interval
2. Delta wave
3. Wide QRS

In presence of pre excitation the diagnosis of ventricular hypertrophy should not be made

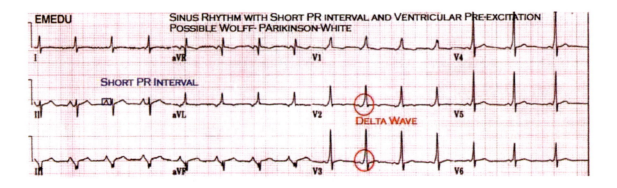

Pericarditis

1. Elevated ST segment and T wave
2. Return close to normal
3. Sharply inverted T wave, isoelectric ST segment

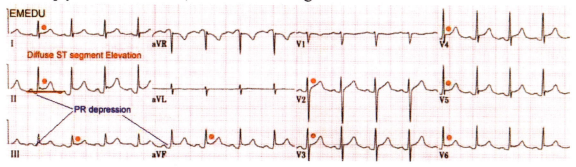

Pericardial effusion

Low voltage QRS < 5 mm in all limb leads

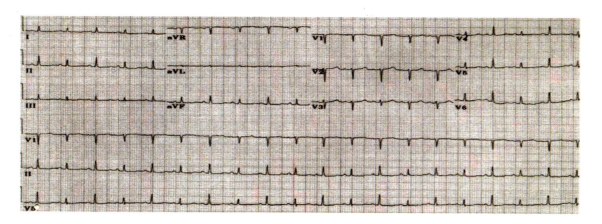

Myocarditis

1. Delayed AV conduction
2. Prolonged QT interval
3. Low magnitude T wave
4. Low voltage QRS < 5 mm in all limb leads

Myocardial infarction

	Limb leads	Pericardial leads
Lateral	I, aVL	V5, V6
Anterior		V1, V2, V3
Anterolateral	I, aVL	V2-V6
Diaphragmatic	II, III, aVF	
Posterior		V1-V3

Phases and changes:

Hyperacute phase	- Elevated ST segment - Deep, wide Q wave
Early phase	- Elevated ST segment - Deep, wide Q wave - Diphasic T wave
Late phase	- Deep, wide Q wave - Sharply inverted T wave
Resolving phase	- Deep, wide Q wave - Normal T wave

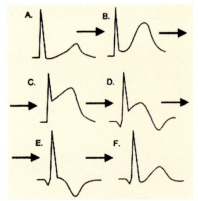

Evolution of Acute myocardial infarction

Electrolyte disturbances

Hypercalcemia:
1. Short ST segment
2. Short QT interval

Hypercalcemia:
1. Prolonged ST segment
2. Prolonged QT interval

Hypokalemia:
1. ST segment depression
2. Flat or diphasic T wave
3. Prominent U wave

Hyperkalemia:
1. Tall T wave
2. Prolonged QRS
3. Prolonged PR interval
4. Disappearance of P wave
5. Wide, bizarre, diphasic QRS (sine wave)
6. Ventricular fibrillation
7. Cardiac arrest

Hyperkalemia ECG changes

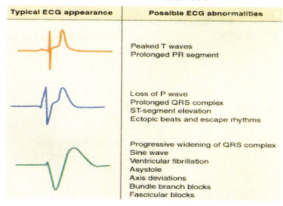

Supraventricular tachycardia

P wave is buried in the T wave of the preceding cycle.

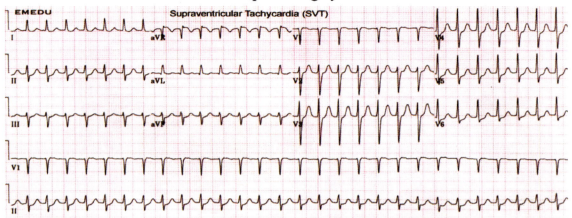

Atrial flutter

Causes:

1. Myocarditis
2. Structural heart disease with dilated atria
3. Acute infectious disease
4. Intra-atrial surgery

Criteria:

1. F wave with "saw tooth" configuration in V1, II, III
2. Atrial rate is 240-360 BPM
3. There is a degree of heart block (2:1, 3:1, etc.)
4. QRS is usually normal

Treatment:

- Short duration: DC cardioversion
- Longer duration: DC postponed while starting warfarin to prevent thromboembolism

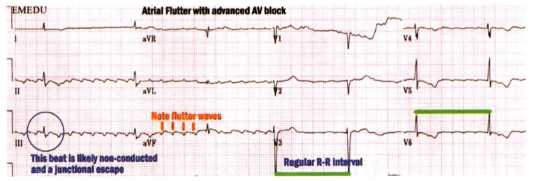

Atrial fibrillation

1. Intra-atrial surgery
2. Structural heart disease

Criteria

1. Atrial rate 350-600 bpm
2. Ventricular response is irregularly irregular
3. QRS is usually normal

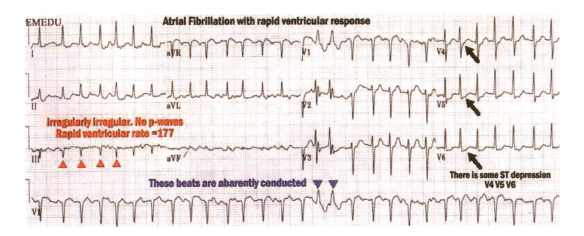

Premature ventricular contraction (PVC)

1. Bizarre, wide QRS occurring before next expected QRS
2. T wave direction opposite to QRS
3. No premature P wave before premature QRS

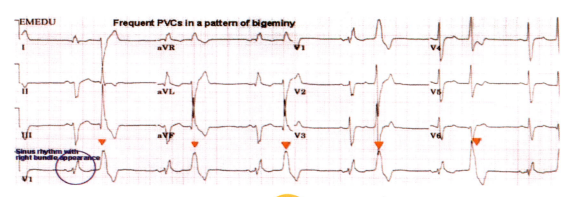

Ventricular tachycardia

3 or more PVCs occurring at rate 120-180 bpm

Causes:

1. Congenital heart disease: fallot tetralogy, TGA
2. Cardiomyopathies
3. Myocarditis
4. Muscular dystrophies
5. Coronary artery abnormalities
6. Cardiac tumors

Treatment:

1. Of the cause
2. Cardioversion
3. Lidocaine
4. Recurrence: propranolol, atenolol

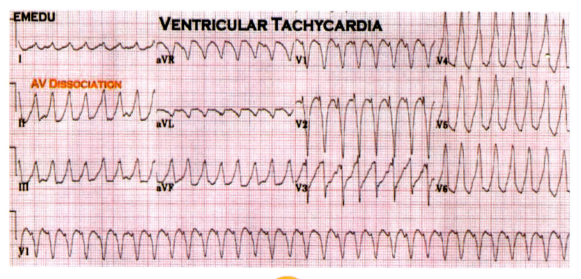

Ventricular fibrillation

1. Bizarre, wide QRS of varying size and configuration
2. Rate is irregular and rapid

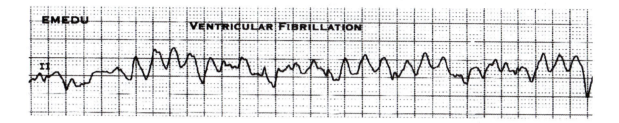

AV block

First degree AV block

Abnormal delay in conduction through AV node

Criteria:

1. Prolonged PR interval
2. Sinus rhythm is maintained
3. No dropped beats
4. QRS is normal

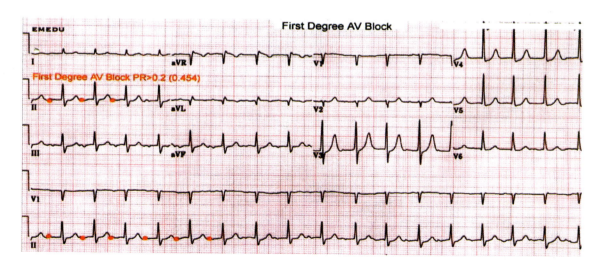

Second degree AV block

Mobitz type I
1. Progressive lengthening of PR interval
2. Dropped ventricular beat over 3-6 cycles
3. Long diastolic pause then the cycle is resumed
4. QRS is normal

Mobitz type II
1. AV conduction is all or none
2. Atrial rate is normal
3. Ventricular rate is dependent on the successfully conducted atrial impulses

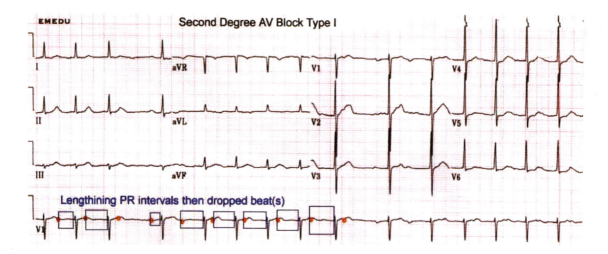

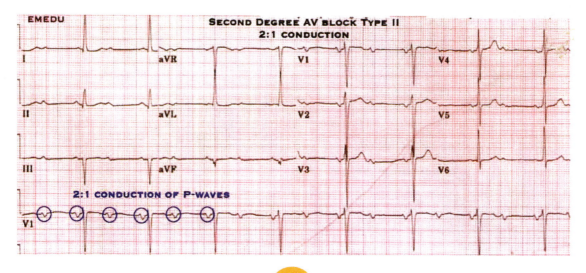

Third degree AV block

1. Atria and ventricles beats independently of one another
2. Atrial rate is regular
3. Ventricular rate is regular but slower
4. QRS is normal

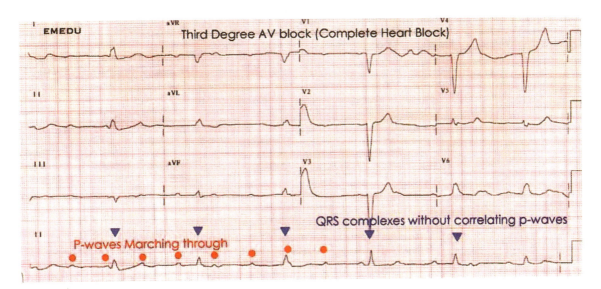

Third degree AV block

1. Atria and ventricles beats independently of one another
2. Atrial rate is regular
3. Ventricular rate is regular but slower
4. QRS is normal

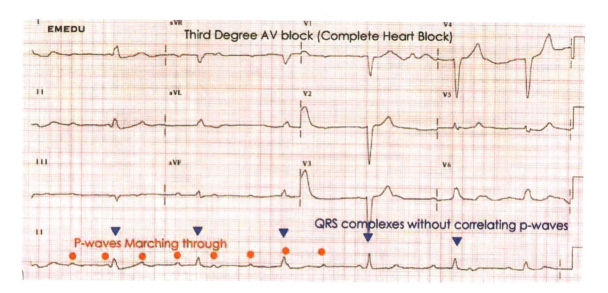

Abbreviations

2-3DPG	diphosphoglycerate	DD	differential diagnosis
AC	air conduction	DI	diabetes insipidus
AD	autosomal dominant	DIC	disseminated intravascular coagulation
ADHD	attention deficit hyperactivity disorder	DIOS	distal intestinal obstruction syndrome
ANA	anti-nuclear antibody	DIP	distal interphalangeal
AP	anteroposterior	DM	diabetes mellitus
AR	aortic regurge	DT	Diphtheria, Tetanus
AR	autosomal recessive	DTaP	Diphtheria, Tetanus, and Pertussis Vaccine
ASD	atrial septal defect	EBV	ebstein barr virus
ATN	acute tubular necrosis	ECG	electrocardiograph
AVSD	atrioventricular septal defect	ECMO	extracorporeal membrane oxygenation
BC	bone conduction	EEG	electroencephalograph
BMA	bone marrow aspirate	EMG	electromyography
BMI	body mass index	ER	emergency room
BMT	bone marrow transplantation	FEV	forced expiratory volume
BP	blood pressure	FFA	free fatty acid
BPD	broncho-pulmonary dysplasia	FISH	fluorescent in situ hybridization
CAH	congenital adrenal hyperplasia	FSH	follicle stimulating hormone
CBC	complete blood count	FVC	forced vital capacity
CHD	congenital heart disease	GH	growth hormone
CHO	carbohydrate	GHRH	growth hormone releasing hormone
CLD	chronic lung disease	GIT	gastrointestinal tract
CMV	cytomegalovirus	GnRH	gonadotrophin releasing hormone
CNS	central nervous system	GSD	glycogen storage disease
COA	coarctation of aorta	GU	genitourinary
COPD	chronic obstructive pulmonary disease	HAART	highly active antiretroviral therapy
CP	cerebral palsy	HiB	haemophilus influenza
CPK	creatine phosphokinase	HIE	hypoxic ischemic encephalopathy
CRH	corticotrophin releasing hormone	HSM	hepatosplenomegaly
CRP	C - reactive protein	IBD	inflammatory bowel disease
CTX	cyclophosphamide	ICP	intracranial pressure
CVS	cardiovascular system	IDDM	insulin dependent diabetes mellitus
CXR	chest x-ray	INH	isoniazid

IPJ	interphalangeal joint	PS	pulmonary stenosis
IPV	inactivated poliomyelitis vaccine	PT	prothrombin time
IUGR	intra-uterine growth retardation	PTH	parathormone
IVH	intraventricular hemorrhage	PTT	partial thromboplastin time
IVIG	intravenous immunoglobulin	PUBS	percutaneous umbilical artery blood sample
JIA	juvenile idiopathic arthritis	PVL	periventricular leukomalacia
JVP	jugular venous pressure	RAST	radioallergosorbent test
LABA	long-acting beta agonist	RES	reticuloendothelial system
LCH	langerhans cell histiocytosis	RF	rheumatoid factor
LH	luteinizing hormone	ROP	retinopathy of prematurity
LHRH	luteinizing hormone releasing hormone	RSV	respiratory syncytial virus
LL	lower limb	S1	first heart sound
LLSE	lower left sternal edge	S2	second heart sound
LN	lymph node	SCA	sickle cell anemia
MCADD	Medium-chain acyl-CoA dehydrogenase deficiency	SIDS	sudden infant death syndrome
MCT	medium chain triglycerides	SOB	shortness of breath
MCUG	micturating cystourethrogram	TB	tuberculosis
MIF	Mullarian inhibitory factor	TGA	transposition of great arteries
MMR	mumps-measles-rubella	TOF	tetralogy of fallot
MPJ	metacarpophalangeal	TPN	total parental nutrition
MR	mitral regurge	TSH	thyroid stimulating hormone
MS	mitral stenosis	UCD	urea cycle defects
MSUD	maple syrup urine disease	UL	upper limb
NEC	necrotizing enterocoitis	ULSE	upper left sternal edge
NGT	nasogastric tube	URTI	upper respiratory tract infection
NPO	nothing per oral	US	ultrasound
NSAIDs	non-steroidal anti-inflammatory drugs	UTI	urinary tract infection
OA	organic acidemia	UVB	ultraviolet B
ORS	oral rehydration solution	VCR	vincristine
PCP	pneumocystis pneumonia	VF	ventricular fibrillation
PCR	polymerase chain reaction	VMA	vanillylmandelic acid
PDA	patent ductus arteriosus	VSD	ventricular septal defect
PEFR	peak expiratory flow rate	VT	ventricular tachycardia
PIP	proximal interphalangeal	VUR	vesicoureteral reflux
		WAS	Wiskott Aldrich syndrome

Index

A

Abdominal Examination · 3, 8
Abetalipoproteinemia · 112
Abortion · 93
Achondroplasia · 32
Acid base status · 117
Acidosis · 107, 117, 127, 128, 135, 155
Acrodermatitis enteropathica · 112
Acute post-streptococcal glomerulonephritis · 129
ADHD · 83, 244
Adrenal gland cortex · 170
Adrenal insufficiency · 127, 172
Agammaglobulinemia · 191
Alkalosis · 117, 152
Ambiguous Genitalia · 169
Anaphylaxis · 149, 150, 214
Anorexia Nervosa · 168, 179
Anterior pituitary gland · 164
Arthrogryposis syndromes · 185
AS · 6, 7, 60, 69
ASD · 6, 7, 60, 69, 233, 244
Asthma · 14, 149, 207, 208, 209, 211
Ataxia · 22, 141, 145
Atopic Eczema · 88
Atrial fibrillation · 239
Atrial flutter · 238
Atrial hypertrophy · 231
Audiogram · 76
Audiometry · 76, 78
Audit · 94
Autistic Spectrum Disorder · 81
Autonomy · 51, 92, 93
AV block · 241, 242, 243
AVSD · 227, 244
Axis determination · 227

B

Balloon atrial septostomy · 69
Barlow · 109
Beckwith – Weidemann syndrome 100, 123, 190
Beighton score · 33
Beneficence · 51, 92, 93
Biliary atresia · 159, 160
Bilirubin · 157
Biventricular hypertrophy · 229
Blue Sclera · 8
Bone · 31, 75, 76, 101, 137, 167, 174, 181, 184, 193
Breaking bad news · 46, 48
Breast Feeding Promotion · 102
Bronchiectasis · 14, 62, 211, 212
Bronchiolitis · 206, 211
Bulge test · 27
Bullying · 84, 178

C

Calcium metabolism · 174
Capillary Hemangioma · 87
Cardiac Arrest · 90
Cardiovascular Examination · 3, 5
Carinatum · 12, 13
Cerebellar system · 21
Cerebral Palsy · 11, 22, 79
Chemoprophylaxis · 194, 195
Chemotherapy · 86, 194, 195
Chronic Diarrhea · 137
Chronic fatigue syndrome · 215
Chronic lung disease · 105, 212
Chronic renal failure · 135
Cirrhosis · 143, 154, 161
Clinical Governance · 96
CNS · 3, 17, 27, 56, 105, 128, 140, 142, 143, 152, 167, 170, 180, 192, 244
CNS Examination · 3, 17
COA · 7, 60, 69, 244
Coagulation pathways · 216
Coeliac disease · 137, 176
Collateral ligament test · 28
Confidentiality · 92
Congenital Adrenal Hyperplasia · 171
Congenital Heart Disease · 60
Congenital infections · 202
Conjugated hyperbilirubinemia · 159
Consent · 46, 47
Constipation · 10, 32, 58, 130, 132, 152, 180, 201, 217
Contraception · 93
Cortical sensations · 20
Cover and uncover test · 16, 73, 74
Cow's milk protein intolerance · 113
Cranial Nerve Examination · 3, 15
Crohn's disease · 10
Cushing · 32, 117, 178
Cyanosis · 5, 12, 105, 114, 206, 209
Cystic fibrosis · 11, 14, 98, 117, 127, 137, 154, 158, 159

Cystinosis · *128, 135*

D

Delayed puberty · *168*
Development · *3, 33, 38, 39, 40, 42, 166*
Developmental Dysplasia of the Hip · *109*
Dextrocardia · *62, 229*
Diabetes Insipidus · *165*
Diabetes mellitus · *176*
Digeorge syndrome · *101*
Digitalis · *228*
Dilated Cardiomyopathy · *66*
Down syndrome · *60, 97, 99, 153, 159, 175*
Dyspraxia · *81, 82*

E

ECG · *3, 63, 66, 67, 68, 70, 127, 142, 186, 224, 237, 244*
ECMO · *65, 120, 244*
EEG · *63, 122, 142, 144, 148, 244*
Electrolytes disturbance · *127*
Endocarditis · *5, 29*
Epilepsy · *81, 141, 144, 145, 146*
Erb's Palsy · *110*
Erythema · *8, 79, 161*
Esophageal atresia · *121*
Evidence based medicine · *95*
Excavatum · *12, 13*
Eye Examination · *3, 16*

F

Facial Palsy · *79*
Fanconi syndrome · *128*
Febrile Convulsions · *124*
Fine Motor · *41*
Friedreich's · *22, 141, 213*
Functional abdominal pain · *85*

G

Gait · *22, 27*
Gait examination · *22*
Galactosemia · *77, 98, 118, 123, 128, 159, 173*
Gastroesophageal reflux · *114*
Gastrostomy · *11, 58, 111*
Genitalia · *166, 171*
Genomic imprinting · *100*
GH · *31, 32, 164, 173, 178, 244*
Glasgow coma scale · *147*
Glomerulonephritis · *129*
Glycogen storage disease · *154, 155*
Glycogen Storage Disease · *10*
Goiter · *33, 35, 181, 182*
Gross Motor · *40, 42*
Gynecomastia · *8, 161*

H

Head injury · *146*
Headache · *56, 70, 84, 138, 146, 199, 200, 201, 215*
Hearing · *41, 44, 78, 81, 184, 202*
Heart rate · *225, 226*
Hemolytic disease of Newborn · *106*
Henoch schonlein purpura · *129*
Henoch-Schonlein purpura · *187*
Hepatomegaly · *5, 10, 65, 154, 155*
Herpes simplex virus · *199*
Hirschsprung disease · *153, 217*
HIV · *86, 159, 195, 197, 198*
Hyperkalemia · *127, 228, 229, 237*
Hypermobility · *33*
Hypersensitivity · *149*
Hyperthyroidism · *159, 181*
Hypertrophic Cardiomyopathy · *67*
Hypoglycemia · *119, 152, 155, 173, 190, 200*
Hypothyroidism · *32, 77, 168, 178, 182, 217, 229*

I

IgA Deficiency · *191*
IgA Nephropathy · *129*
Immune · *101, 149, 163, 191*
Infant feeding · *55, 103*
Infection · *60, 65, 66, 77, 88, 103, 104, 122, 129, 137, 175, 177, 191, 192, 193, 197, 205, 206, 211, 212, 245*
Inhaler devices · *210*
Insulin · *127, 170, 173, 175, 177, 178*
Insulin Dependent Diabetes Mellitus · *175*
Interventional Cardiac Catheters · *69*
Intraventricular hemorrhage · *107*
Intussusception · *115*

J

Janeway lesions · *5*
JIA · *183, 245*
Jugular venous pressure · *5, 8, 61*
Justice · *51, 92, 93*
Juvenile idiopathic arthritis · *154, 183*

K

Kawasaki disease · *186*
Kyphoscoliosis · *117, 141, 213*

L

Left bundle branch block · *233*
Left ventricular hypertrophy · *227, 232*
Leishmaniasis · *201*
Liver failure · *29, 143, 162*
Liver transplant · *161, 163*
Long QT syndromes · *230*
Lung function tests · *203*

M

Malaria · *154, 200*
Manoeuvers · *30*
Measles · *141, 192, 199*
Medical error · *46, 49*
Metabolic disorders · *116, 122, 141*
Mobitz type I · *242*
Mobitz type II · *242*
Mucopolysaccharidosis · *32, 67, 77, 124, 213*
Mumps · *199*
Musculoskeletal · *3, 24, 56*
Myasthenia Gravis · *80, 119*
Myocardial infarction · *229, 236*
Myocarditis · *186, 228, 229, 230, 235, 238, 240*

N

Necrotizing enterocolitis · *108*
Neonatal hypoglycemia · *123*
Neonatal seizures · *122*
Nephrotic syndrome · *129, 200*
Neurofibromatosis Type I · *140*
Neuromuscular · *22, 23*
Nocturnal enuresis · *132*
Non-compliant · *46, 50*
Non-maleficence · *51, 92, 93*
Noonan · *31, 67, 80, 227*
Nutritional Assessment · *3, 11*
Nystagmus · *15, 16, 72, 141*

O

Obesity · *30, 178*
Optic nerve pathway · *71*
Ortolani · *109*
Osler's nodules · *5*
Osteogenesis imperfecta · *184, 185, 213*
Osteomyelitis · *188, 193, 201*
Oxygen dissociation curve · *204*

P

Patellar tap · *27*
PDA · *7, 60, 69, 105, 107, 108, 212, 245*
Pericardial effusion · *228, 235*
Pericarditis · *68, 183, 186, 194, 229, 235*
Perthes Disease · *22, 188*
PGALS · *3, 24, 25, 27, 29*
Pneumothorax · *12*
Poisoning · *152*
Polyps · *12*
Portal hypertension · *64, 154, 156, 161*
Portal Vein Obstruction · *10*
Port-Wine Stain · *87*
PR interval · *70, 225, 228, 234, 237, 241, 242*
Precocious puberty · *167*
Premature atrial contraction · *230*
Premature ventricular contraction · *239*
Preterm babies · *105*
Primary ciliary dyskinesia · *14*
PS · *6, 7, 60, 69, 245*
Pseudobulbar Palsy · *79*
Psoriasis · *89, 189*
Psoriatic Arthritis · *189*
Ptosis · *15, 16, 80*
Pulmonary Hypertension · *6, 64, 65*

Q

Q wave · *229, 232, 233, 236*
QRS complex · *228*

R

Radio-femoral delay · *5*
Renal Osteodystrophy · *135, 137*
Renal transplant · *10, 136*
Renal tubular physiology · *126*
Reproductive tract · *166*
Respiratory Examination · *3, 12*
Reviews · *3, 59*
Right bundle branch block · *233*
Right ventricular hypertrophy · *227, 232*
Rubella · *199, 202*
Russell Silver Syndrome · *31, 33*

S

Scars · *10, 35*
School refusal · *84*
Scoliosis · *5, 8, 9, 12, 30, 32, 140, 185*
Screening tests · *98*
Sensory examination · *20*
Septic Arthritis · *193*
Severe combined immunodeficiency · *191*
Short Stature · *3, 30*
Shunt Nephritis · *129*
Sick sinus syndrome · *226*
Sinus arrhythmia · *226*
Sinus bradycardia · *226*
Sinus rhythm · *225, 241*
Sinus tachycardia · *226*
Situs inversus · *5, 62*
SLE · *60, 119, 129, 135*
Social · *41, 44, 57, 81, 83, 84, 132*
Sore throat · *205*
Speech · *41, 78, 82, 147, 190*
Splenomegaly · *5, 10, 154, 156*
Splinter hemorrhage · *5*
Squints · *73*
Sternotomy · *7*
Stridor · *114, 212, 214*

Sudden infant death syndrome · *125*
Supraventricular tachycardia · *238*
Syncope · *63, 70*

T

Tall Stature · *3, 33*
TB · *14, 136, 159, 172, 192, 193, 194, 195, 245*
Telangiectasia · *141*
Thomas test · *28*
Thyroid · *3, 33, 34, 67, 119, 176, 178, 181, 182, 215, 217*
Tics · *18, 139*
TOF · *7, 60, 245*
Trachea-esophageal fistula · *121*
Transfusion · *104, 151, 197*
Tuberculosis · *68, 194, 195, 196*
Tuberous sclerosis · *142*
Turner · *31*
Typhoid fever · *201*

U

Umbilical artery catheterization · *104*
Unconjugated hyperbilirubinemia · *158*
Urinary tract infection · *130, 134*

V

Vaccination · *56, 86, 202, 212*
Ventricular fibrillation · *237, 241*
Ventricular tachycardia · *240*
Vesicoureteral Reflux · *134*
Vision · *16, 39, 41, 55, 56, 105*
VSD · *7, 60, 245*

W

Weber and Renee Test · *75*
William's syndrome · *189*
Wilson's disease · *18, 141, 143, 154, 159*
Wolf-Parkinson-White syndrome · *70, 234*

References

- Robert M. Kliegman, Bonita M.D. Stanton, Joseph St. Geme, Nina F Schor, Richard E. Behrman. Nelson Textbook of pediatrics, 19th edition 2011.

- Mark Beattie, Mike Champion. Essential Revision Notes in Paediatrics for the MRCPCH, 2nd edition 2006.

- Simon Bedwani, Christopher Anderson, Mark Beattie. MRCPCH Clinical: Short Cases, History Taking and Communication Skills, 3rd edition 2011.

- Stanley T. Zengeya, Tiroumourougane, Serane V. The MRCPCH Clinical Exam Made Simple, 2011.

- Myung K. Park, Warren G. Guntheroth. How to read pediatric ECGs, 4th edition 2006.

- Rebecca Casans, Milthilesh Lal. Communication Scenarios for the MRCPCH and DCH clinical Exams, 2nd edition 2011.

- ECG images: ECG interpretations for emergency physicians, http://www.emedu.org/ecg/

- Neurology examination images: OSCE Skills, http://www.osceskills.com/e-learning/modules/neurology/

- Sensory examination images: Matt's training resources, http://nothinbutapeanut.com/?page_id=577

- Musculoskeletal, PGALS, Joint examination images: http://www.arthritisresearchuk.org/

- Beighton score image: Korean Academy of Rehabilitation Medicine, Ann Rehabil Med. 2013 Dec; 37(6):832-838. English.

- Optic nerve pathway image: https://commons.wikimedia.org/wiki/File:Wiley_Human_Visual_System.gif

- Weber & Rinne test image: http://pixshark.com/rinne-test.htm

- Audiogram images: Hearing loss in children, https://entcare.wordpress.com/tag/hearing/

- Hemangioma image: Arch Soc Esp Oftalmol Vol.87 No. 12 Madrid DIC. 2012

- Port wine stain image: http://www.babyrashclinic.com/rash-in-babies-face-due-to-port-wine-stain/

- Evidence based medicine image: EBM Pyramid and EBM Page Generator, Produced by Jan Glover, David Izzo, Karen Odato and Lei Wang.

- Genomic imprinting image: http://genetics4medics.com/prader-willi-syndrome.html

- ECMO image: transferred from de:Datei:Ecmo schema.jpg, by Author; Jürgen Schaub. de:User:Mr.Flintstone

- Gastrostomy image: Fortunato, J. E. and C. Cuffari (2011). "Outcomes of percutaneous endoscopic gastrostomy in children." Curr Gastroenterol Rep 13(3): 293-299.

- Tracheoesophageal fistula: https://www.med-ed.virginia.edu/courses/rad/gi/esophagus/congen02.html

- Wilson disease image: Silberang/Yang, Color Atlas of Pathophysiology, [2000]

- Bilirubin metabolism image: http://www.hepatitis.va.gov/

- Hypersensitivity reaction image: http://cnx.org/contents/14fb4ad7-39a1-4eee-ab6e-3ef2482e3e22@7.28.

- Renin angiotensin system image: http://renalfellow.blogspot.com/2009/08/basic-review-renin-angiotensin.html

- Bone and calcium metabolism image: Vitamin D and Cardiovascular Disease, Ibhar Al Mheid, Riyaz S. Patel, Vin Tangpricha, Arshed A. Quyyumi. DOI: http://dx.doi.org/10.1093/eurheartj/eht166 3691-3698 First published online: 10 June 2013

- Calcium metabolism image: naoyuki T, Nobuyuki U., vitamin D endocrine system and osteoclasts. Bonekey reports (2014) 3, article number: 495 (2014).

- Lung function tests image: https://www.studyblue.com

I have done every effort to contact copyright owners to obtain permission to reproduce copyright materials. Having overlooked any material unintentionally or by mistake, I would be pleased to set the necessary arrangements to be dealt with in the next reprints.

Go Pass

First Edition 2015

ISBN-13: 9781515246602

ISBN-10: 1515246604

"NADIA HAMMAD"